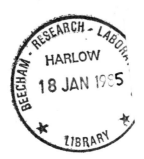

Drug Design: Fact or Fantasy?

Based on the Proceedings of the Third Rhône-Poulenc
Round Table Conference entitled "Drug Design: Fact or Fantasy?"
held in Eastbourne from 3-5 November, 1982.

Drug Design:
Fact or Fantasy?

Edited by

G. JOLLES

Rhône-Poulenc Santé
Paris, France

K.R.H. WOOLDRIDGE

May and Baker Ltd
Dagenham, Essex
Great Britain

1984

ACADEMIC PRESS

A Subsidiary of Harcourt Brace Jovanovich, Publishers

London   Orlando   San Diego   San Francisco   New York
Toronto   Montreal   Sydney   Tokyo   São Paulo

ACADEMIC PRESS INC. (LONDON) LTD
24/28 Oval Road
London NW1

United States Edition published by
ACADEMIC PRESS INC.
(Harcourt Brace Jovanovich, Inc.)
Orlando, Florida 32887

British Library Cataloguing in Publication Data
Drug design.
　　1. Pharmacology—Congresses
　　I. Jolles, Georges　　II. Wooldridge, K.R.H.
　　615'.1　　RM300

　　ISBN 0-12-388180-3
　　LCCCN 83-70976

Printed in Great Britain by
Galliard (Printers) Limited, Great Yarmouth

List of Participants

Andrews P.R.   Professor, Dean, School of Pharmaceutical Chemistry, Victorian College of Pharmacy Ltd., 381 Royal Parade, Parkville, Victoria 3052, Australia.

Ashford A.   Biological Research Manager, May and Baker Ltd., Dagenham, Essex, Great Britain.

Ashton M.J.   Chemical Research, May and Baker Ltd., Dagenham, Essex, Great Britain.

Barreau M.   Département de Chimie Pharmaceutique, Rhône-Poulenc Recherches, Centre Nicolas Grillet, Vitry-sur-Seine, France.

Blanchard J.C.   Département de Pharmacologie, Rhône-Poulenc Recherches, Centre Nicolas Grillet, Vitry-sur-Seine, France.

Blondel J.C.   Direction Scientifique, Rhône-Poulenc Santé, Paris-La Défense, France.

Bost P.E.   Directeur des Programmes et des Projets de Recherches, Rhône-Poulenc Santé, Paris-La Défense, France.

Bouchaudon J.   Département de Chimie Pharmaceutique, Rhône-Poulenc Recherches, Centre Nicolas Grillet, Vitry-sur-Seine, France.

Bowden K.   Department of Chemistry, University of Essex, Colchester, Great Britain.

Caillard C.   Adjoint au Directeur du Département de Pharmacologie, Rhône-Poulenc Recherches, Centre Nicolas Grillet, Vitry-sur-Seine, France.

Caton M.P.L.   Chemical Research Manager, May and Baker Ltd., Dagenham, Essex, Great Britain.

Cattier-Humblet C.   Laboratoire de Pharmacochimie Moléculaire, Centre de Neurochimie du C.N.R.S., Strasbourg, France.

Chapman R.F.   Assistant Chemical Research Manager, May and Baker Ltd., Dagenham, Essex, Great Britain.

Choplin F.   Service de Documentation, Rhône-Poulenc Recherches, Centre de Recherches des Carrières, St. Fons, France.

Clementi S.   Professor, Dipartimento di Chimica, Universita di Perugia, Via Elce di Sotto, 10-06100, Perugia, Italy.

Cotrel C.   Département de Chimie Pharmaceutique, Rhône-Poulenc Recherches, Centre Nicolas Grillet, Vitry-sur-Seine, France.

Dearden J.C.   School of Pharmacy, Liverpool, Great Britain.

Debarre F.   Direction Scientifique, Rhône-Poulenc Santé, Paris-La Défense, France.

Depaire H.   Service d'Analyse Structurale, Rhône-Poulenc Recherches, Centre Nicolas Grillet, Vitry-sur-Seine, France.

Dreux C.   Professeur, Université René Descartes, (Paris V), Vice-Président de SPECIA, Paris, France.

Dubosc Y.   Chef du Service Documentation, Rhône-Poulenc Recherches, Centre Nicolas Grillet, Vitry-sur-Seine, France.

Farge D.   Adjoint au Directeur des Recherches Chimiques Pharmaceutiques, Rhône-Poulenc Recherches, Centre Nicolas Grillet, Vitry-sur-Seine, France.

Fenton G.   Chemical Research, May and Baker Ltd., Dagenham, Essex, Great Britain.

Fujita T.   Professor, Department of Agricultural Chemistry, Kyoto University, Kyoto 606, Japan.

Guinot F.   Directeur Général Adjoint, Rhône-Poulenc Santé, Paris-La Défense, France.

Hansch C.   Professor, Seaver Chemistry Laboratory, Pomona College, Claremont, California 91711, USA.

Iddon B.   Department of Chemistry and Applied Chemistry, University of Salford, Salford, Great Britain.

James C.   Département de Chimie Pharmaceutique, Rhône-Poulenc Recherches, Centre Nicolas Grillet, Vitry sur Seine, France.

Jeambourquin R.   Directeur du Centre de Recherches de Vitry, Rhône-Poulenc Recherches, Centre Nicolas Grillet, Vitry-sur-Seine, France.

Jollès G.   Directeur Scientifique, Rhône-Poulenc Santé, Paris-La Défense, France.

Julou L.   Directeur des Recherches Biologiques Pharmaceutiques, Rhône-Poulenc Recherches, Centre Nicolas Grillet, Vitry-sur-Seine, France.

Loveless A.   Biological Research, May and Baker Ltd., Dagenham, Essex, Great Britain.

Lunt E.   Chemical Research, May and Baker Ltd., Dagenham, Essex, Great Britain.

McFadzean J.A.   Director of Research, May and Baker Ltd., Dagenham, Essex, Great Britain.

Marshall G.R.   Professor, Department of Physiology and Biophysics, Washington University School of Medicine, 660 South Euclid Avenue, St. Louis, Missouri 63110, USA.

Messer M.   Directeur des Recherches Chimiques et Biochimiques Pharmaceutiques, Rhône-Poulenc Recherches, Centre Nicolas Grillet, B.P. 14 F 94400 Vitry-sur-Seine, France.

Moutonnier C.   Département de Chimie Pharmaceutique, Rhône-Poulenc Recherches, Centre Nicolas Grillet, Vitry-sur-Seine, France.

Ollis D.   Professor, Department of Chemistry, The University, Sheffield, Great Britain.

Palfreyman M.N.   Chemical Research, May and Baker Ltd., Dagenham, Essex, Great Britain.

Phillipson R.F.   Resources Manager Pharmaceutical Research, May and Baker Ltd., Dagenham, Essex, Great Britain.

Ponsinet G.   Département de Chimie Pharmaceutique, Rhône-Poulenc Recherches, Centre Nicolas Grillet, Vitry-sur-Seine, France.

Rabin B.R.   Professor, Department of Biochemistry, University College, London, Great Britain.

Ramsden C.A.R.   Corporate Chemistry Unit, May and Baker Ltd., Dagenham, Essex, Great Britain.

Riche C.   Institut de Chimie des Substances Naturelles du C.N.R.S., Gif-sur-Yvette, France.

Roques B.P.   Professeur, Département de Chimie Organique, U.E.R. des Sciences Pharmaceutiques et Biologiques, Université René Descartes, 4 Avenue de l'Observatoire, 75270 Paris Cedex 06, France.

Salmon J.   Chemical Research, May and Baker Ltd., Dagenham, Essex, Great Britain.

Smith C.   Chemical Research, May and Baker Ltd., Dagenham, Essex, Great Britain.

Stevens M.   Professor, Department of Pharmacy, University of Aston in Birmingham, Birmingham, Great Britain.

Tomlinson E.   Professor, Department of Pharmacy, University of Amsterdam, Amsterdam, The Netherlands.

Trouet A.   Professeur, Faculté de Médecine, Université Catholique de Louvain, International Institute of Cellular and Molecular Pathology, 75 Avenue Hippocrate, B-1200 Brussels, Belgium.

Walsh R.J.A.   Chemical Research, May and Baker Ltd., Dagenham, Essex, Great Britain.

Warburton D.   Assistant Chemical Research Manager, May and Baker Ltd., Dagenham, Essex, Great Britain.

Wermuth, C.G.   Professeur, Laboratoire de Chimie Organique, Faculté de Pharmacie, Université Louis Pasteur, 74 Route du Rhin, B.P. 10, 67048 Strasbourg Cedex, France.

Whalley W.B.   Professor, Pharmaceutical Chemistry, The School of Pharmacy, University of London, London, Great Britain.

Withnall M.   Biochemical Research, May and Baker Ltd., Dagenham, Essex, Great Britain.

Wold S.   Chemometrics Research Fellow, Research Group for Chemometrics, Umeå University, S-901 87 Umeå, Sweden.

Woolridge K.R.H.   Pharmaceutical Research Manager, May and Baker Ltd., Dagenham, Essex, RM10 7XS Great Britain. Visiting Professor, City University and University of Essex.

Preface

*"L'inconnaissable n'est
que de l'inconnu provisoire"*

This volume contains the Proceedings of the Third Rhône-Poulenc Round Table, held at Eastbourne on the south coast of England in November 1982.

The aim of this meeting was to determine to what extent modern tools offered by computers, mathematics or new biological theories could now be effectively used to achieve the old dream fostered by chemotherapists, i.e. to design a new drug by logical thought and calculation and, as far as possible, not to rely on chance.

"What is unknowable is but temporarily unknown".

"If only man willingly collects and implements the appropriate means, then ignorance fades away, as a shadow from sunlight. Only material obstacles build a screen between the truth and ourselves. Human ignorance is not hopeless: with time and money, man may acquire and learn everything."

This credo assigned to scientists by Grassé in his essay on the natural history of man* is quite reassuring for the future of drug design which, undoubtedly, will be outstanding. But today, in 1983, what is the situation, Fact or fantasy?

The objective of the Eastbourne Round Table was to seek an answer from top specialists in various methodologies of drug design who met with scientists from the pharmaceutical industry who are faced every

* P. P. Grassé (1971) 'Toi, ce petit Dieu" p. 227, Albin Michel, Paris.

day with practical problems. The former successively reviewed their personal approaches and the latter explained the philosophy which they adopted after long and concrete experience. In this book, the reader will in no way discover recipes but an overall evaluation. He will confront his own convictions and, with a view to his own choices, will find the basic parameters of drug design and the evaluation obtained after many discussions. In fact, this book not only contains the presentations of the contributors but also the main discussions of the subgroups in which the participants expressed themselves more freely and reached sometimes differing conclusions which were finally discussed by the full conference.

It is our objective that this book should provide a better understanding of the knowledge acquired and of the shortcomings in the field of drug design and that it should give rise to positive cross-fertilization between optimists and pessimists for improved efficacy in research. It is our hope that by helping research scientists in their strategic considerations, it will contribute to the discovery of new and valuable drugs.

G. Jolles and K. R. H. Wooldridge

Acknowledgements

It is our real pleasure to thank warmly all the contributors and participants who agreed to attend the meeting and to work actively together, in a friendly atmosphere of free discussion. We are especially thankful to the four chairmen of the Round Table: Professors Rabin, Tomlinson, Whalley and Ollis.

We are particularly indebted to Drs Blondel and Phillipson who assisted us most efficiently in the organization of the meeting and to Drs Bowden, Julou, McFadzean, Messer and Professor Wermuth for their advice and help in preparing the programme of the conference.

We want further to express our gratitude to our colleagues of the Rhône-Poulenc Group of Companies who assisted us in the editorial task of reviewing, preparing and finalizing the text of the various contributions and discussions: M. Barreau, J.C. Blondel, M. Caton, R. Chapman, F. Choplin, E. Lunt, A. Loveless, R. Phillipson, C. Ramsden, C. Smith, R. Walsh and M. Withnall.

Finally we wish to acknowledge the efficiency of Dr Mary Firth in charge of the transcription of the discussions, of the translators of the French presentations Miss Eiglier and Mrs Tantet, and of Miss Cox who took care of our guests.

The expert assistance of the staff of Academic Press Inc. (London) Ltd. in producing this volume was greatly appreciated.

G. Jolles and K. R. H. Wooldridge

Opening Remarks

Dr G. JOLLES

It is my honour and privilege to open this morning the third Round Table Conference organized by the Rhône-Poulenc Group of Companies, a meeting for which we have chosen the deliberately provocative title: "Drug Design: Fact or Fantasy?"

For the past few years, it has been our objective to examine at regular intervals a scientific topic of current interest by organizing round tables with university specialists and research staff from the industry. The purpose of such meetings was to carry out a synthetic approach to the topics in order to prepare the way for new research strategies and to stimulate new activities in that particular field.

It was in this way that, in 1978, we achieved an overview of the Pharmacology of Immunoregulation and, in 1980, tried to determine the Future of Antibiotherapy and Antibiotic Research. Today, we wish to concentrate on a different issue, an issue which often gives rise to passionate arguments and directly concerns our everyday work.

"Drug Design: Fact or Fantasy?": this title actually requires two explanations: what do we mean by drug design and why the question mark?

A few weeks ago, I attended an International Symposium at which research executives of some large pharmaceutical companies were discussing many of their problems. At one point, we were trying to find the French or German equivalent to "drug design", but in the end it appeared that fairly long paraphrases were required to express this same concept. In order to avoid any problem of semantics during the present meeting for this unique and very concise expression, I should like to state that, in our opinion, it corresponds to rational methodologies which give access to a new drug either through the noblest pathway, namely total innovation, or through the more tangible pathway, optimization.

On the other hand, why in fact do we question the reality of drug design?

Is it a dispute between the ancients and moderns; between conservative and progressive tendencies? Definitely not. Yet everything has its share of reality and dream: in the best champagne, we must distinguish the foam, which we see, from the wine, which we drink, and what is expected of a good drug research scientist is that he acts intelligent not that he looks intelligent.

As a matter of fact, I am now close to the point where I may be blamed for trying to advocate a pre-established opinion, and this is exactly what I should like to avoid during this symposium. There is no pre-established opinion to back up in favour of fact or fantasy: drug design exists; otherwise what would be the point of such a programme, and how could we have managed to gather such a panel of personalities all of whom have accepted to talk about their methodologies and their techniques.

But what are the real possibilities of application today; what are the domains in which drug design may be most fruitful; what are the actual limitations which must be overcome to make it perform better tomorrow? These are the real questions to which we trust you will help provide the answers.

The review to which we shall proceed together consists of two distinct parts. In the first part, specialists of the major techniques proposed to design new drugs or to optimize them will explain the main features of their areas of activity and the results of their research. Furthermore, two of our experts will present, under two different aspects, the view of research scientists who have been faced for many years with the problem of discovering new drugs. In the second part, all the participants will meet in syndicates in order to facilitate discussions on a very broad basis of the various theories and methodologies, with special emphasis on their individual experiences.

During the final session, a general and constructive evaluation of the discussions and of the answers to our questions will be worked out with a view to conferring practical usefulness to this Round Table which, we hope, will be rewarding for all of us.

We have excluded, intentionally, from our programme all presentations of results which would be too restrictive, and of course, although the example of an original research work may be welcome to illustrate the recommended methods, we hope that the discussions will concentrate less on the technical aspects of each methodology than on its potential as a tool for the discovery of new drugs.

It is, in fact, on drug design potential, strategy and, may I say, philosophy, that we wish to lay stress and I am certain that our meeting will be successful if we can meet this goal.

I should like to thank now all our speakers, some of whom have come from far away, and all our university guests who accepted our invitation and give of their precious time to be with us. I know that everybody will be interested to see how the individual areas can be integrated into the very broad spectrum of possible approaches to drug design.

I want to thank, also, all those who participated in the organization of this Round Table, my colleague Dr Wooldridge with whom I have been working hand in hand and Drs Phillipson and Blondel who took care of the general technical arrangements. We really tried to make this meeting a symbol of the excellent cooperation between the centres of the Health Division in France and those of May and Baker.

The discovery of a new drug is indeed an extremely difficult task. Maybe it was imprudent of us to adopt this shining expression, "Drug Design", from people who are really designers, who design aeroplanes, cars, equipment: they know exactly what they are aiming for; they are aware of most of the parameters involved in their project; they can calculate.

The crucial difference in drug research is that we do not dominate all the parameters as far as we have even identified them and, therefore, work under a serious handicap. For this reason, many scientists now-adays still believe in the virtues of intelligent screening as a major tool for innovation, and among them are some of the most successful ones. Others have total faith in the available rational approaches; they cannot stand even to hear about screening and practice the most evident disdain for an alliance with serendipity.

What then is the truth about drug design at this time? Well, we have prepared the dossier; we have provided the experts; there will be prosecutors and defendants either for fact or for fantasy; but the judges will be you.

Please, let it be a fair trial.

Contents

Session I

1 Targeting of Drugs

**A. TROUET, D. DEPREZ-DE CAMPENEERE,
R. BAURAIN and Y.-J. SCHNEIDER**

*Université Catholique de Louvain, International
Institute of Cellular and Molecular Pathology,
75 Avenue Hippocrate, B – 1200 Brussels, Belgium*

The concept of drug targeting, which was already described more than 80 years ago by Paul Ehrlich is very simple and straightforward. It starts from the observation that most of the pharmacological agents and drugs are not very selective with regard to their cellular sites of action and present therefore various side-effects which are neither expected nor needed. Targeting involves the concept that the selectivity of drugs can be enhanced and their toxic side-effects decreased by associating them with carriers which, pharmacologically inactive themselves, will convey the drugs selectively towards their target cells (Trouet, 1978). Although this concept is very simple in theory, it took more than 50 years before first attempts were made to put it into practice.

We would like to discuss here the theoretical and practical implications of drug targeting and to illustrate them with some of the results obtained in our research group while attempting to apply this concept to the chemotherapy of cancer and of protozoal diseases. We believe that, to be efficient, the drug, the carrier and the link between these entities should fulfil a well defined set of criteria. The carrier should be able to transport the drug from the site of its administration to its target cell and interact with this latter as selectively as possible. It has been overlooked too much that the drug should remain inactive as long

DRUG DESIGN: FACT OR FANTASY
ISBN 0.12.388180.3

as it is linked to its carrier and as long as it is transported in the blood-stream and extracellular spaces. As a corollary to this requirement, one needs a mechanism by which the drug will be reactivated after inter-action of the carrier with its target. The link between the drug and the carrier should thus be stable in the bloodstream and extracellular spaces but be reversible after interaction with the target cell.

The targeting effect of the carrier molecules has to rely on a specific interaction with cellular binding sites, such as receptors or antigens. Two different classes of carriers can be considered depending on the pericellular or intracellular localization of their recognition sites. If the specific receptors are intracellular, the carrier itself should permeate through cell membranes which will exclude any molecules such as peptides and proteins like antibodies. Moreover, an intracellular drug activation mechanism triggered by the interaction of the carrier and its receptor has to be available. This latter requirement makes it very dif-ficult to target drugs via carriers selective for intracellular sites, since such an activation mechanism is not available according to our present knowledge of cell biology. Attempts have, however, been made to link antitumour drugs such as alkylating agents to carriers such as hormones (Wall *et al.*, 1969). The targeted drug remained, however, active when linked to its carrier with the consequence that the targeting effect was mainly lost because the drug was able to interact with many non-target cells during its transport to the cancer cells.

The potentially most interesting carriers will interact with specific binding sites present at the surface of the target cells. These carriers should not be able to permeate through the cell membranes and there-fore the carrier-linked drug should be inactive against non-target cells. Another major advantage of this class of carriers is the possibility that, as we have proposed in 1972 (Trouet *et al.*, 1972), the drug can be activated after endocytosis by the target cell of the drug-carrier con-jugate and its subsequent intracellular processing by the acid hydrolases of the lysosomal compartment (Fig. 1). Indeed, if the carrier and the link between the drug and the carrier have been chosen appropriately, the drug can be released from its carrier through hydrolysis by lysosomal enzymes; this hydrolysis being triggered by the endocytosis of the drug–carrier conjugate.

The criteria which have to be fulfilled by an ideal lysosomotropic drug–carrier conjugate can be summarized as follows:

1) the carrier should be selective for the target cell surface, be endo-cytosed upon interaction with its receptor or binding site and reach the lysosomal compartment;
2) the carrier itself should be degraded by lysosomal enzymes in order to avoid lysosomal overload;

DRUG TARGETING AND ACTIVATION

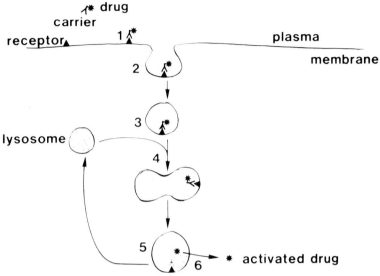

FIG. 1   Mechanism of entry and of activation of a drug–carrier conjugate taken up by receptor-mediated endocytosis. The drug–carrier conjugate (𝒜*) binds to its receptor (1), the cellular membrane invaginates (2) and engulfs the conjugate (3), the endocytic vacuole fuses then with a lysosome (4) where the conjugate or the link between the carrier and the drug is split by lysosomal hydrolases or the acid pH (5), the activated drug exits from the lysosome to reach its intracellular site of action (6).

3) the carrier should finally be non-immunogenic and be able to permeate through the anatomical barriers, such as the capillary walls, which separate the administration site from the target cells;
4) the drug should be resistant to lysosomal enzymes and acid pH in order not to be inactivated after endocytosis and intralysosomal processing;
5) the drug should also be able to cross the lysosomal membrane upon release if it is expected to act in extralysosomal cell compartments;
6) finally, the link between the drug and the carrier should remain stable in the bloodstream and extracellular spaces while being sensitive to lysosomal enzymes or acid pH to allow the release of the drug in an active form.

Several classes of carriers have been advocated and used experimentally to transport a large variety of antitumour and anti-infectious drugs. Without enumerating and detailing all of them here, we have to mention first erythrocytes (Ihler, 1979) and platelets (Ahn *et al.*, 1978) in which drugs can be incorporated. Their drug entrapment capacity is, however, poor as well as their blood stability, and their selectivity is restricted mainly towards cells of the reticulo-endothelial system. A whole variety of synthetic or semi-synthetic and complex carriers has also been tested such as nanoparticles (Speiser, 1976), microspheres (Kramer, 1974) and liposomes (Gregoriadis, 1976). For the nanoparticles and microspheres there remains the largely unsolved problem of poor enzymatic degradability while for all of them, and in particular the liposomes, the degree of selectivity which can be achieved is hindered through a preferential uptake by the cells of the reticulo-endothelial system. However, recently the selectivity of liposomes was improved by associating them with glycolipids (Lau *et al.*, 1981). We proposed earlier the possibility of using DNA as a carrier for intercalating antitumour drugs such as daunorubicin (DNR) and doxorubicin. These complexes, however, being of non-covalent nature tend to dissociate in the bloodstream (Trouet *et al.*, 1979). They have moreover, no known cell selectivity and their use is restricted to drugs which bind reversibly to double stranded DNA.

The most promising carriers seem to be proteins such as antibodies, peptide hormones or glycoproteins because they possess a very wide variety of specificities, are degradable and can be non-immunogenic. In view of these considerations, we developed, as a first step, a general method for linking the antitumour drug DNR to proteins which would fulfil the criteria required by the targeting concept as discussed above (Trouet *et al.*, 1982). This work was done in close collaboration with Dr. Ponsinet and Dr. Messer of the Centre de Recherches de Vitry of Rhône-Poulenc.

We had shown previously (Trouet *et al.*, 1972) that DNR is resistant *in vitro* to lysosomal hydrolases and acid pH. On the other hand, DNR possesses an amino group on its daunosamine moiety which is very well suited for establishing an amide type of linkage with carboxylic side chains of proteins. This amino group is, however, essential for the activity of DNR and has therefore to be restored after lysosomal hydrolysis of the amide linkage. We prepared such covalent conjugates of DNR and bovine serumalbumin (SA), used as a model protein. It very soon became obvious that it was impossible to release any active DNR from this conjugate by *in vitro* incubation in the presence of lysosomal enzymes. Suspecting that this inability to release intact DNR could be due, at least partly, to steric hindrance, we prepared DNR−SA conjugates incorporating a spacer-arm (1 to 4 amino acids) between DNR and the protein (Fig. 2).

The reversibility of these conjugates was then tested by incubation in the presence of lysosomal enzymes at 37°C and pH 5.5 and monitoring the release of intact DNR by means of HPLC and fluorometry (Baurain *et al.*, 1979). From the data of Table 1, it can be seen that no

CONJUGATION OF DNR TO A PROTEIN

with a spacer arm

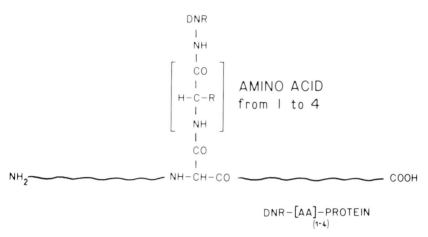

DNR−[AA]−PROTEIN
(1-4)

FIG. 2   Structure of the daunorubicin−serumalbumin conjugates. Daunorubicin is linked to serumalbumin either directly or via an oligopeptidic spacer arm composed of 1 to 4 amino acids.

TABLE 1

Influence of the peptide spacer-arm length on the release by lysosomal peptidases of DNR linked to bovine serumalbumin

Conjugates	% DNR released after		
	1 h	4 h	10 h
SA−DNR	0	1.0	2.6
SA−(aa)$_1$−DNR	0.6	2.3	5.0
SA−(aa)$_2$−DNR	2.0	5.0	8.0
SA−(aa)$_3$−DNR	24.4	47.0	59.5
SA−(aa)$_4$−DNR	21.1	55.3	74.1

The conjugates were incubated at 37°C and pH 5.5 in the presence of 5 mM cysteine and 0.5 mg/ml of purified lysosomal fraction from rat liver. The amount of DNR released was determined by HPLC and fluorometry and expressed in percent of the linked drug.

DNR is released from the DNR−SA direct conjugate while some DNR appears in the incubation medium when one amino acid or a dipeptide is intercalated. However, between 60 and 80% respectively of the conjugated DNR was liberated when a tri- and a tetra-peptide spacer-arm was used. The tetra-peptide spacer-arm used is illustrated in Fig. 3 and consists of leucyl−alanyl−leucyl−alanine. Although some flexibility

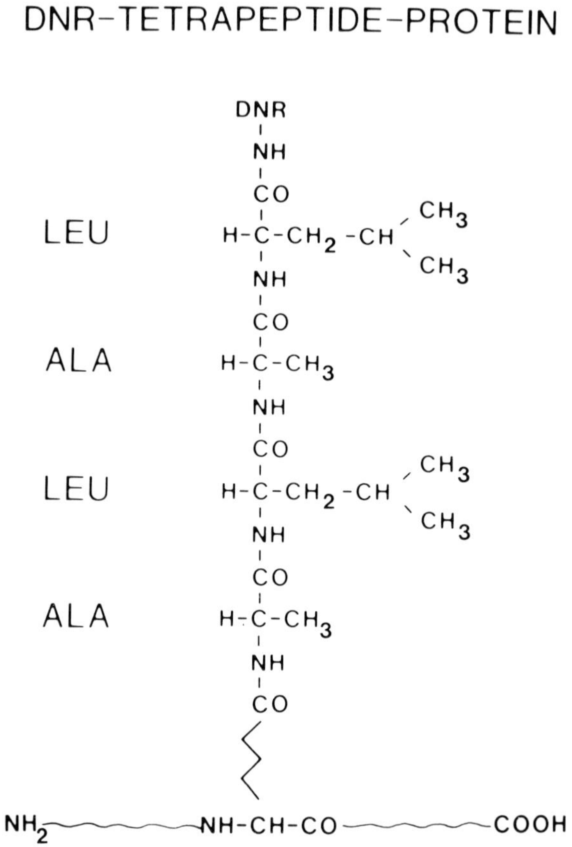

DNR-TETRAPEPTIDE-PROTEIN

```
                        DNR
                        |
                        NH
                        |
                        CO
                        |            CH3
   LEU              H-C-CH2 -CH
                        |            CH3
                        NH
                        |
                        CO
                        |
   ALA              H-C-CH3
                        |
                        NH
                        |
                        CO
                        |            CH3
   LEU              H-C-CH2 -CH
                        |            CH3
                        NH
                        |
                        CO
                        |
   ALA              H-C-CH3
                        |
                        NH
                        |
                        CO
                        
                        <

NH2~~~~~~~~~~~~NH-CH-CO~~~~~~~~~COOH
```

FIG. 3   Structure of the daunorubicin–tetrapeptide–serumalbumin conjugate.

is allowed in the nature of the two or three last amino acids it is important to have a leucyl amino acid adjacent to DNR since amongst various amino acid derivatives of DNR tested, leucyl–DNR was the most extensively and rapidly hydrolysed into DNR by lysosomal enzymes (Masquelier *et al.,* 1980).

Several reports on the linking of DNR to proteins have been made but they indicated either that the conjugates were inactive *in vivo* or that not enough precautions were taken to remove from the conjugates any DNR which was not linked covalently but adsorbed tightly on to the proteins.

The stability in the bloodstream of the DNR–tetrapeptide–SA conjugate was checked during an *in vitro* incubation in the presence of serum, and *in vivo* after i.v. injection into mice. As illustrated in Fig. 4, the conjugate is very stable in the bloodstream since no free DNR could

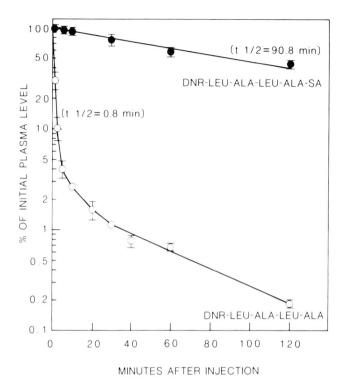

FIG. 4 Plasma disappearance of daunorubicin–tetrapeptide free or linked to serumalbumin, after i.v. injection into mice. DBA2 mice received i.v. DNR–leu–ala–leu–ala–SA (●) or DNR–leu–ala–leu–ala (○) at a dose corresponding to 7 mg DNR/kg. Serumalbumin was ^{14}C-labelled before linking to DNR tetrapeptide. TCA insoluble radioactivity was followed in the plasma and drugs were analyzed by HPLC and fluorometry. Mean ± S.D. of 2 separate assays are given.

be detected. The plasma half-life of the conjugate was 90.8 min as compared with 0.8 min for that of free DNR – tetrapeptide.

The activity of the DNR conjugates was determined *in vivo* using experimental L1210 murine leukaemia. The results given in Table 2 clearly illustrate the correlation between the *in vitro* and *in vivo* experiments. The DNR – SA conjugate without a spacer-arm and that with one amino acid have no chemotherapeutic activity. The conjugate with an intercalated dipeptide arm has an activity comparable to that of free DNR while the conjugates with the tri- and tetra-peptide spacer-arm display a very striking antileukaemic effect which overshadows completely that of free DNR. The enhanced chemotherapeutic activity of the DNR – tri- or tetra-peptide – SA conjugates is most probably not the result of a targeting effect of SA but rather the consequence of the altered pharmacokinetic characteristics of the conjugated drug which

TABLE 2

Chemotherapeutic activity of the DNR–serumalbumin conjugates on murine L1210 leukaemia[a]

	Molar ratio DNR/PROTEIN	Dose mg/kg per day in PROTEIN	Dose mg/kg per day in DNR	ILS[b] %	Number of survivors on day 30
					Total number of mice
DNR	—	—	2	39	5/91
	—	—	5	6	0/52
	—	—	7.5	7	0/8
SA–DNR	11.6	51	5	9	0/9
	11.6	77	7.5	9	0/6
SA–(aa)$_1$–DNR	12.1	49	5	6	0/10
	12.1	74	7.5	6	0/10
SA–(aa)$_2$–DNR	14.4	41	5	30	0/10
	14.4	62	7.5	33	0/10
SA–(aa)$_3$–DNR	17.1	35	5	>200	6/10
	20.8	43	7.5	>211	8/10
SA–(aa)$_4$–DNR	15.1	39	5	107	4/10
	15.0	40	5	>211	7/10
	15.1	59	7.5	>211	6/10
	15.0	59	7.5	>211	10/10
SA	—	59	—	−6	0/16

[a] 10^4 L1210 cells were inoculated i.p. on day 0 into DBA$_2$ mice. Drugs were given i.p. on days 1 and 2.

[b] ILS: increase in life span.

is probably kept for a much longer time in contact with the leukaemic cells inside the peritoneal cavity.

In the development of targeted antitumour drugs there now remains the other major problem of finding carrier molecules which will selectively interact with tumour cells. The molecules which could be used as antitumour drug carriers can be subdivided into five classes. It should be kept in mind that not all of these proteins are capable of interacting exclusively with tumour cells. However, very significant progress could be achieved in cancer chemotherapy by the use of carriers which interact with both cancer cells and some normal cell types but which prevent the drug penetrating into those normal cells, such as those of the bone marrow, gastro-intestinal tract or myocardium, which are very sensitive to the action of antitumour drugs in general, and anthracyclines in particular.

1) Antibodies directed against tumour specific antigens. However, up to now, no demonstrative evidence has been reported in favour of the existence of such antigens in humans.

2) Antibodies directed against tumour associated antigens. These are antigens which although not specific for cancer cells, are mainly found in tumour cells during the postnatal life. They are mainly foetal or embryonic antigens reappearing during cancer transformation such as α-foetoprotein, and carcino embryonic antigen (CEA) for example. On the other hand, immunoglobulin secreting leukaemic cells also possess idiotypic immunoglobulins at their surface. Antibodies to their idiotype will therefore only interact with these clonal antigens and thus be specific for the cells.

3) Antibodies to tissue specific or organotypic antigens. A good example would be antibodies directed to specific antigens of the mammary epithelial cells. These antigens seem to be shared by mammary tumour cells both from the primary tumour and metastases (Ceriani *et al.*, 1980). Such antibodies would be very useful in the treatment of disseminated breast cancer.

4) Peptide hormones. A good example is β-melanotropin, recognized by malignant melanoma cells (Varga *et al.*, 1977).

5) Glycoproteins which interact with hepatocytes or with macrophages as a function of the nature of their terminal carbohydrate moieties. For example, desialylated fetuin with terminal galactose residues interacts selectively with hepatocytes and some hepatoma cells (Schwartz *et al.*, 1981).

As far as antibodies are concerned, it is important to realize that they can only function as carriers if they interact with antigens present at the cell surface and if they are endocytosed. On the other hand, the antibody preparation should be pure. Polyclonal antibodies should therefore be purified by immunoadsorbtion or monoclonal antibodies be used.

We would also like to point out some of the difficulties which could be encountered when using antibodies as carriers for antitumour drugs. Cell surface antigens from the tumour cells can be found as free antigens circulating in the bloodstream. This seems to be the case for tumour associated antigens such as α-foetoprotein and CEA. One should be aware that in this case the drug carrying antibodies will react with the circulating antigens before reaching their targets. This problem could, however, be overcome by eliminating these antigens first by administration of drug-free antibodies or by extracorporeal immunoadsorbtion.

Tumour cells and more precisely leukaemic antigens have been shown to undergo antigenic modulation upon administration of specific monoclonal antibodies (Ritz et al., 1982). The cell surface antigens seem to disappear from the cell surface upon interaction with antibodies. These antigens are probably endocytosed and this problem could accordingly be overcome by the use of drug associated antibodies which would be able to kill the cells before modulation of the antigens.

One of the major question marks with regard to the use of antibodies as carriers resides in the possible antigenic heterogeneity of the tumour cell population. The main question is whether all the cells of the primary tumour and its metastases possess the antigens or the receptors used for targeting. There is a lot of discussion about the heterogeneity of tumour cell population and there is no doubt that this heterogeneity exists with regard to the metastasizing potential of the cells and with regard to their drug responsiveness (Hart et al., 1981).

Another important limitation which could result from the use of antibodies in human chemotherapy is their immunogenicity since they are animal proteins. This problem will, however, most probably be circumvented in the next few years by the use of monoclonal antibodies of human origin which are presently being developed in several laboratories.

In addition to its use in cancer chemotherapy, the drug targeting concepts can also be applied to chemotherapy of intracellular infections. Experiments in chemotherapy of the exoerythrocytic (i.e. hepatocytic) stage of murine malaria caused by *Plasmodium berghei* allowed us to demonstrate the validity of the drug targeting concept in general and to apply our conjugation method developed for DNR to the antimalarial drug, primaquine (PQ) (Trouet et al., 1983).

The first stages of infection by Plasmodium involve the hepatocytes, into which the sporozoites inoculated by the mosquitoes penetrate and develop into schizonts which in turn invade the circulating red blood cells. The treatment of the exoerythrocytic stages of malaria is difficult because the few active drugs, amongst them PQ, cannot be used to their full extent because of toxic side effects.

Since glycoproteins with a terminal galactose residue react specifically with receptors on the hepatocytic surface, and are endocytosed and digested inside the lysosomes (Hartford *et al.*, 1982), we have linked PQ via a tetrapeptide spacer-arm to one such glycoprotein: desialylated fetuin (asialofetuin).

In vitro digestion experiments in the presence of lysosomal enzymes showed that PQ could not be released from the proteins in intact form, as monitored by HPLC and UV photometry unless a peptide spacer-arm was inserted between the amino group of PQ and the protein carboxylic side chains. As a control, we prepared PQ–asialofetuin conjugates, in which the galactose residues were masked by extensive succinylation of the amino groups of the protein. These two conjugates and free PQ were injected i.v. into mice inoculated i.v. 3 hours before with *Plasmodium berghei* sporozoites. PQ, either free or conjugated, was given at a dosage of 25 mg/kg which corresponds to the maximum tolerated dose for free PQ. The chemotherapeutic experiments illustrated in

TABLE 3

Antimalarial activity of primaquine and primaquine–asialofetuin conjugates[a]

DRUG	Dose[b] (mg/kg)	ILS[c] (%)	LTS/N[d]
Controls	–	0	0/223
PQ	6.25	46	0/6
	12.5	58	11/33
	15.0	166	10/23
	20.0	110	25/55
	25.0	>320	50/94
	30.0[e]	– 91	2/9
PQ–(aa)$_4$–ASF[f]	6.25	100	1/12
	10.0	170	5/12
	12.5	160	7/16
	15.0	>400	7/12
	20	>400	5/6
	25	>400	12/12
PQ–(aa)$_4$–Succ.–ASF	6.25	26	0/7
	12.5	68	0/7
	25	68	1/7
	35	>163	4/7
	50	>163	5/8

[a] Drugs were given intravenously 3 hours after i.v. inoculation of the *P. berghei* sporozoites to male TB$_{ESP}$ mice.
[b] Doses are expressed in mg PQ diphosphate equivalents/kg body weight.
[c] ILS: increase in life span.
[d] Long-term survivors over the number of treated mice.
[e] Toxic dose.
[f] ASF: asialofetuin.

Table 3 indicate that free PQ cures about 50% of the infected animals. The same dose of PQ conjugated to the hepatotropic glycoprotein, however, cures 100% of the mice while most of the therapeutic effect is lost when PQ is administered conjugated to the succinylated asialofetuin. These results illustrate clearly that targeting of drugs can be achieved *in vivo*.

Conclusion

As a general conclusion, drug targeting could be the source of very important progress in cancer chemotherapy but could also help to solve the major problems which still restrict or prevent chemotherapy of intracellular infections such as those caused by protozoa and viruses. The concept could also be adapted to the treatment of parasitic diseases. In this latter case, it would be necessary to study the selective appetite of these multicellular organisms and to attach drugs to their preferred foodstuff. One can think finally of the development of selective immunosuppressors by linking cytotoxic drugs to antigens or antigen epitopes. These antigen–drug conjugates could then be used to kill the population of lymphocytes which are capable of binding them selectively.

References

Ahn, Y.S., Byrnes, J.J., Harrington, W.J., Cayer, M.L., Smith, D.S., Brunskill, B.E. and Pall, L.M. (1978). *N. Engl. J. Med.* **298**, 1101–1107.

Baurain, R., Deprez-de Campeneere, D. and Trouet, A. (1979). *Cancer Chemother. Pharmacol.* **2**, 11–14.

Ceriani, R.L., Sosoki, M., Peterson, J.A. and Black, E.W. (1980). *In* "Cell Biology of Breast Cancer" (C.M. McGrath, M.J. Breuman and M.A. Reich, eds), pp. 33–56. Academic Press, New York.

Gregoriadis, G. (1976). *N. Engl. J. Med.* **295**, 704–710.

Hart, I.R. and Fidler, I.J. (1981). *Biochem. Biophys. Acta* **651**, 37–50.

Hartford, J. and Ashwell, G. (1982). *In* "The Glycoconjugates", Vol. IV (M.I. Horowitz, ed.), pp. 27–55. Academic Press, New York.

Ihler, G. (1979). *In* "Drug Carriers in Biology and Medicine" (G. Gregoriadis, ed.), pp. 129–153. Academic Press, London, New York.

Kramer, P.A. (1974). *J. Pharm. Sci.* **63**, 1646–1647.

Lau, E.H., Cerny, E.A. and Rahman, Y.E. (1981). *Br. J. Haematol.* **47**, 505–518.

Masquelier, M., Baurain, R. and Trouet, A. (1980). *J. Med. Chem.* **23**, 1166–1170.

Ritz, J. and Schlossman, S.F. (1982). *Blood* **59**, 1–11.

Schwartz, A.L., Fridovich, S.E., Knowles, G.G. and Lodish, H.F. (1981). *J. Biol. Chem.* **257**, 4230–4237.

Speiser, P. (1976). *Prog. Colloid Polym. Sci.* **59**, 48–57.

Trouet, A. (1978). *Eur. J. Cancer* **14**, 105–111.

Trouet, A., Deprez-de Campeneere, D. and de Duve, C. (1972). *Nature (London) New Biol.* **239**, 110–112.

Trouet, A., Deprez-de Campeneere, D., Baurain, R., Huybrechts, M. and Zenebergh, A. (1979). *In* "Drug Carriers in Biology and Medicine" (G. Gregoriadis, ed.), pp. 87–105. Academic Press, New York.

Trouet, A., Masquelier, M., Baurain, R. and Deprez-de Campeneere, D. (1982). *Proc. Natl. Acad. Sci. U.S.A.* **79**, 626–629.

Trouet, A., Pirson, P., Baurain, R. and Masquelier, M. (1983). In "Antimalarial Drugs" (W. Peters and W.H.G. Richards, eds), Springer–Verlag, Berlin, in press.

Varga, J.M., Asato, N., Lande, S. and Lerner, H.B. (1977). *Nature (London)* **267**, 56.

Wall, M.E., Abernath, G.S. and Carkoll, F.I. (1969). *J. Med. Chem.* **12**, 810–818.

Discussion

Chairman: Professor Rabin

Professor Rabin

It occurs to me that tumours are immunologically very distinct. Do you not think, Professor Trouet, that this will create a very great problem in designing systems?

Professor Trouet

The problem is that in human cancer not enough is known about what I call the "tumour-specific" antigens. There is a big question mark about it. Do tumour-specific antigens really exist? There is, however, much evidence in the literature about the existence of tumour-associated antigens being shared by different cells of the same tumour cell population.

My major concern is the tumour cell population heterogeneity. Do metastases of any given tumour share all the antigens that are found in each primary tumour? We have developed a methodology, and what we would like to do – what we are trying to do now – in human cancer (because it is useless to develop carriers for mouse leukaemia and we have to go to humans) is to see how far tumour-associated antigens, and tissue-specific antigens in the case of mammary cancer, are shared by all the cells of a primary tumour and by the metastases. This is the key – but I cannot provide an answer yet.

Professor Rabin

It sounds as though you have a very high level of optimism that the methodology will work reasonably effectively. Are you thinking in terms of using human monoclonal antibody systems?

Professor Trouet

It is well-known that the development of human monoclonal antibodies is still in its infancy, so I think that we will have to work first with murine monoclonal antibodies.

I am optimistic, and I think it is possible to be optimistic if we are also very cautious, knowing all the pitfalls – and even being aware of other pitfalls that cannot be foreseen. The problem, I think, is that too many people have tried to go too fast in this field by linking antitumour drugs and in fact we did the same several years ago. All the aspects have to be considered and we should go into the practical applications only when we are sure about all the factors involved.

Professor Rabin

The other problem, of course, is what normal cell is used to compare with the tumour cell. Of course, tumours have to originate from stem cells, and these are impossible to obtain in quantity.

Professor Trouet

Yes, but it depends on the tumour. For example, for the tumours originating from the haematopoietic system there is of course the problem of the stem cells. Again, I know of several monoclonal antibodies directed against leukaemic antigens in humans. This is not our work, but the people who have done it claim that several of these antibodies are shared by leukaemic cells and are absent in normal haematopoietic stem cells − as far as can be seen on bone marrow smears, for example.

The problem is different in solid tumours. If we consider breast cancer, for example, the reason why we are very interested is because there we have tissue-specific antigens and there is no need to worry about the stem cells.

Professor Tomlinson

There are three orders of drug targeting:

1) First-order targeting, whereby the carrier takes the drug to a particular organ.

2) Second-order targeting, whereby the carrier is directed towards a particular diseased part of an organ.

3) Third-order targeting, which Professor Trouet has described so elegantly today, where the carrier takes the drug molecule into the cell, by whatever mechanism that may be hypothesised.

What is Professor Trouet's opinion on second-order targeting, in particular on the use of particular materials which can take drug molecules to the diseased site, and thereupon release their drug in a pharmaceutically controlled manner without a specific recognition event? I know that it is not so elegant bio-chemically, but pharmaceutically it is much more simple, and of course it is much more applicable to many different types of drug molecules. We could, in fact, envisage a carrier which would be a universal carrier, at least for a particular group of molecules, because there would not have to be a specific recognition event.

Professor Trouet

I think that you do not refer to a question of drug targeting but to a question of prodrugs: that is why I did not include this aspect in my presentation.

The main problem is that we have to think about the method of activation. The activation mechanism is very often overlooked − I mean the activation mechanism that has to be used in drug targeting or in prodrugs in order to have the drug released at a given site, either selectively or non-selectively.

We have to think about enzymes, about the physiological conditions, pH and so on, which will enable a drug linked to a carrier to be released at a given site. Therefore, it is very important in this concept, too, that we have a drug−carrier conjugate which is stable as long as it does not interact with the activation system. This is why I do not agree with the people working on liposomes or DNA (as we did) because these drugs are released before arriving at their site. This is true both for the drug targeting and for the prodrug concept. I agree, though, that there are many possibilities.

Dr Withnall
Professor Trouet mentioned briefly that immunogenicity may be a problem. Is this a major problem, say, with immunoglobulins as carriers, and is it possible that we are in a better situation with molecules, such as the asialoglycoproteins, for transport to the liver?

Professor Trouet
In the antibody field, we have the problem of whether it will be possible to have human monoclonal antibodies – otherwise we shall have to resort to murine monoclonal antibodies, and hope that these immunological problems will not be too great: we can assume that, because antitumour drugs are usually immunosuppressive. This question of selective immunosuppression may already apply with the immunoglobulins that are injected with the cytotoxic drugs. There is a fair possibility that the immunologically competent cells which will recognize this immunoglobulin will be killed by the daunorubicin that is carried. This should be tested.

As for the glycoproteins, we have ongoing experiments in the malaria field where serumalbumin with galactose residues is used: we hope that they will provide us with the adequate answers as to this immunogenicity problem.

Professor B. Roques
What is the reason for the importance of the leucine side chain in the vicinity of the drug?

Professor Trouet
The probable reason is the following: if daunorubicin is linked directly to the protein, the lysosomal enzymes are releasing a daunorubicin–amino acid derivative, which is not further cleavable by lysosomal enzymes. Therefore, the last amino acid linked to daunorubicin is no longer cleaved. Rhône-Poulenc prepared several amino acid derivatives of daunorubicin, which we tested: the first step was to see whether they were transformed into daunorubicin in the presence of lysosomal enzymes. It transpired that the leucyl derivative was the most sensitive derivative to this cleavage.

Professor Stevens
Professor Trouet's results with the daunorubicin conjugate with the four-spacer were very striking in comparison with daunorubicin in the L1210 test. He attributed that enhanced activity to pharmacokinetic reasons. Was the activity of the conjugate investigated against L1210 resistant to the parent drug?

Professor Trouet
No.

Professor Stevens

So, in fact, it has not been proved to be pharmacokinetic reasons. There could be an entirely novel antitumour species.

Professor Trouet

It is not a novel pharmacological species because the conjugate itself is inactive. It has to be degraded and it has to release daunorubicin in order for it to be active.

Professor Stevens

How can that be known if it has not been tested against the daunorubicin-resistant cell lines?

Professor Trouet

Daunorubicin-resistant cell lines would not provide an answer. If the conjugate was active (which is possible), against the daunorubicin-resistant cell lines, that would mean that the mechanism of daunorubicin resistance is at the cell surface on the membrane, but not at the lysosomal membrane. For example, I could consider that this conjugate would be active on drug-resistant L1210 leukaemia if the drug does not get into the cell normally, because the membrane is impermeable to the free drug, but that if the conjugate gets into the lysosomes, the lysosomal membrane is permeable to the free drug.

I think it is an interesting experiment which should be done — but not for that reason.

2 The Role of QSAR in Drug Design

T. FUJITA

*Department of Agricultural Chemistry,
Kyoto University, Kyoto 606, Japan*

Introduction

In recent years, various quantitative structure–activity relationship (QSAR) procedures have been developed covering diverse fields of biologically active compounds including medicinal drugs and pesticides. Among them, the Hansch approach has been most widely and effectively used (Hansch and Fujita, 1964; Hansch, 1976). It assumes that the potency of a certain biological activity exerted by a series of congeneric compounds is expressible in terms of a function of various physicochemical parameters of the compounds. If the function could be formulated showing that certain physicochemical properties are favourable to the activity, the structural modifications which enhanced such properties would be expected to generate compounds of potent activity. Thus, a number of attempts have been made to apply the Hansch approach to the designing of compounds having an optimized structure among congeners (Cramer *et al.*, 1979; Unger, 1980; Wooldridge, 1980; Martin, 1981).

In Japan, as in other countries, the utility of the QSAR procedures has gradually come to the attention of practising chemists in industry during the last decade, and successful applications to the designing of new drugs, mostly by means of the Hansch approach, have accumulated recently (Fujita, 1978, Fujita, 1982). In this article, two examples, one

DRUG DESIGN: FACT OR FANTASY
ISBN 0.12.388180.3

for a quinolone carboxylic acid antibacterial agent (Koga, 1982) and the other for an N-benzylacylamide herbicide (Kamoshita and Kirino, 1982), are presented to show the present state of drug design research in Japan, as well as to review the overall role of the Hansch QSAR procedure in drug design.

Design of a Novel Quinolone Carboxylic Acid Antibacterial Drug, AM-715

Nalidixic acid (1) is the first member of an antibacterial drug family sharing a common γ-pyridone-β-carboxylic acid structure (Lesher *et al.*,

1962). Although it has been clinically used against infections due to most of the Gram-negative bacteria, it is only very weakly effective against most of the Gram-positive and *Pseudomonas* bacteria. Thus, a number of efforts have been made to enhance the antibacterial activity, as well as to expand the antibacterial spectrum, by modification of its structure. Oxolinic acid (2) and pipemidic acid (3) are noteworthy examples among

a number of analogues thus developed. Oxolinic acid was characterized by its potent antibacterial activity and pipemidic acid was marked by its broader antibacterial spectrum, including its effect upon *Pseudomonas* (Albrecht, 1977).

Under these circumstances several years ago, Koga and his co-workers of Kyorin Pharmaceutical Company, Tokyo, began their attempt to develop compounds having not only more potent activity and a broader spectrum, but also lower oral toxicity as well as higher stability to metabolism than any other nalidixic acid analogues known at that time (Koga *et al.*, 1980). They selected 4-quinolone-3-carboxylic acid (4) as

4

the reference compound, since its analogues can be prepared more easily than those having such polyazanaphthalene ring systems as those in nalidixic and pipemidic acids.

They synthesized analogues having various substituents inserted at different positions systematically (Koga *et al.*, 1980). They determined the minimum inhibitory concentration (m.i.c. in M) against *Escherichia coli* NIHJ JC-2 for each compound, since it was observed that the activity against this bacterium roughly parallels that against Gram-negative rod-shaped bacteria including *Pseudomonas* (Koga *et al.*, 1980). The structure−activity relationship was first analysed stepwise in terms of substituent effects at each position and the analyses were then extended to the multiply substituted analogues (Koga, 1982). For each of the analyses, correlations with such physicochemical parameters as π, σ_m, σ_p, F, R, E_s, MR and STERIMOL values (Hansch and Leo, 1979) were examined and the statistically best equation was selected. The E_s values were taken from a combined set including the original Taft values and those for hetero-atom substituents estimated according to Kutter and Hansch by (averaged) van der Waals radius (Kutter and Hansch, 1969). The π values were those from the monosubstituted benzene series (Hansch and Leo, 1979).

For derivatives where R^6 in (4) is varied (H, F, Cl, NO_2, Br, Me, OMe and I), but R^1 is fixed to be Et, and for which the log (1/m.i.c.) value ranges between 3.5 and 5.2, Eq. 1 was derived.

$$\log(1/\text{m.i.c.}) = -3.318[E_s(6)]^2 - 4.371[E_s(6)] + 3.924 \qquad [1]*$$
$$\phantom{\log(1/\text{m.i.c.}) = } (0.59) (0.85)$$

$$n = 8 \quad s = 0.108 \quad r = 0.989$$

---

* In this and the following equations, n is the number of compounds used in the regression analysis, s is the standard deviation and r is the correlation coefficient. The figures in parentheses are the 95% confidence intervals.

In this equation, the E_s value of OMe is not that given by Kutter and Hansch, but is taken as that of Et. For NO_2, the value estimated from the half-thickness in terms of the van der Waals dimension is used (Kutter and Hansch, 1969). Equation 1 shows that the effect of R^6 on the activity is mainly steric in nature as far as these eight substituents are concerned. There is an optimum steric dimension in terms of E_s ($= -0.66$), which is located in between those of F and Cl.

For substituent effects at the 8-position, Eq. 2 was formulated for seven derivatives (4: R^1 = Et; R^8 = H, F, Cl, Me, OMe, Et and OEt), the activity index of which varies between 2.5 and 5.0.

$$\log(1/m.i.c.) = -1.016[B_4(8)]^2 + 3.726[B_4(8)] + 1.301 \qquad [2]$$
$$(0.46) \qquad\qquad (2.04)$$

$$n = 7 \quad s = 0.221 \quad r = 0.978$$

Equation 2 shows that the effect of R^8 is also steric. Since the "maximum" width STERIMOL B_4 parameter best represents the steric effect of substituents at this position, these substituents seem to be extended in the direction opposite to that of the R^1 ($=$ Et) substituent. The optimum B_4 value is 1.83, which is close to that of Cl.

At the 2-position of the pipemidic acid (3) skeleton which corresponds to the 7-position of the quinolone carboxylic acid (4), such substituents as alkoxy, alkylthio, alkylamino and dialkylamino (including pyrrolidinyl and piperazinyl) have been known to favour activity, and the favourable effect has been considered to be due to their electron-donating properties (Minami, 1975). The result for eight compounds (4: R^1 = Et; R^7 = H, NO_2, Ac, Cl, Me, OMe, NMe_2 and piperazinyl) was not necessarily in accordance with this earlier point of view. Although the introduction of substituents into the 7-position enhances the activity 10- to 30-fold, the physicochemical factors responsible for the effect were not clear. In terms of the $\log(1/m.i.c.)$ value, the activity varies only from 5 to 5.5 for compounds with substituents ranging from electron-withdrawing NO_2 to electron-donating NMe_2.

Representing the effect of R^7 with an indicator variable $I(7)$, they combined the results for the three sets of "mono" substituted derivatives and derived Eq. 3.

$$\log(1/m.i.c.) = -3.236[E_s(6)]^2 - 4.210[E_s(6)] + 1.358 \, I(7)$$
$$(0.89) \qquad\qquad (1.26) \qquad\qquad (0.40)$$

$$-1.024[B_4(8)]^2 + 3.770[B_4(8)] + 1.251 \qquad [3]$$
$$(0.32) \qquad\qquad (1.43)$$

$$n = 21 \quad s = 0.205 \quad r = 0.978$$

Equation 3 predicts that multiply-substituted derivatives having optimized substituents at each of the 6, 7 and 8 positions [$E_s(6) = -0.65$, $I(7) = 1$ and $B_4(8) = 1.84$] show a log (1/m.i.c.) value of 7.5, which corresponds to their being about ten times more active than oxolinic acid (2).

In an attempt to prove the above prediction, as well as to elaborate the quantitative correlation, the Kyorin workers prepared a number of such multiply-substituted derivatives. For the compounds where $R^6 =$ F, but R^7 is varied from such simple substituents as Cl, Me and NMe_2, to such heterocyclic groups as pyrrolidinyl, piperazinyl and variously N'-substituted piperazinyl, covering the activity range of 3.9 − 6.6, Equation 4 was formulated.

$$\log(1/\text{m.i.c.}) = -0.244\,[\pi(7)]^2 - 0.675\pi(7) - 0.705\,I(7N\text{-CO}) + 5.987 \quad [4]$$
$$(0.05) \qquad\qquad (0.15) \qquad\quad (0.27)$$

$$n = 22 \quad s = 0.242 \quad r = 0.943$$

$I(7N\text{-CO})$ is an indicator variable for such 7-N-heterocyclic substituents as N'-acylpiperazinyl and 4-carbamoylpiperidinyl. The presence of this term indicates that carbonyl functions as a part of the 7-N-substituent lower the activity. In Eq. 4, the 7-unsubstituted compound (4: $R^1 =$ Et, $R^7 =$ H) is not included, since the activity of this compound is about 0.8 log unit lower than that expected from Eq. 4. The reason for this is not obvious, but the effect of R^7 substituents, except for that of the carbonyl function, seems to be composed of two parts. One can be expressed by an $I(7)$ term, the coefficient of which is about 0.8, and the other is determined by the hydrophobicity. The optimum π value is estimated as 1.38. The π value of the piperazinyl group is − 1.74 (calculated from the experimentally determined log P values for the 7-piperazinyl and unsubstituted analogues), and that of the N'-methyl-piperazinyl group is estimated as − 1.24. These values are close to the optimum.

In the above analyses, the R^1 substituent was fixed as Et. As the R^1 substituents in addition to Et, such substituents as $CH=CH_2$, OMe, CH_2CH_2F and CH_2CHF_2, which are sterically similar to Et, were known to be favourable for activity (Albrecht, 1977). Derivatives were prepared in which $R^6 =$ F and $R^7 =$ piperazinyl, but R^1 is varied (Me, Et, $CH=CH_2$, Pr, allyl, hydroxyethyl, benzyl and dimethylamino-ethyl), and the results were analysed for substituent effect to give Eq. 5,

$$\log (1/\text{m.i.c.}) = -0.492[L(1)]^2 + 4.102[L(1)] - 1.999 \quad [5]$$
$$(0.18) \qquad\qquad (1.59)$$

$$n = 8 \quad s = 0.126 \quad r = 0.955$$

where L is the STERIMOL length parameter. There is an optimum length for the R^1 substituent at about 4.2 which coincides with that of Et (L = 4.11).

At this point, it is conceivable that the best substituents at each position are likely to be R^1 = Et, R^6 = F or Cl, R^7 = piperazinyl or N'-methylpiperazinyl and R^8 = Cl or Me. By combining the results for some additional polysubstituted derivatives with those for compounds included in Eqs 3, 4 and 5 as well as with the value deleted from the formulation of Eq. 4, they finally derived Eq. 6 for 71 compounds.

$$\log(1/\text{m.i.c.}) = -0.362[L(1)]^2 + 3.036[L(1)] - 2.499[E_s(6)]^2$$
$$\phantom{\log(1/\text{m.i.c.}) = }(0.25) \qquad (2.21) \qquad (0.55)$$

$$-3.345[E_s(6)] + 0.986 \ I(7) - 0.734 \ I(7N\text{-}CO)$$
$$(0.73) \qquad\quad (0.24) \qquad\quad (0.27)$$

$$-1.023[B_4(8)]^2 + 3.724B_4(8) - 0.205[\Sigma\pi(6,7,8)]^2$$
$$(0.23) \qquad\qquad (0.92) \qquad\quad (0.05)$$

$$-0.485\Sigma\pi(6,7,8) - 0.681\Sigma F(6,7,8) - 4.571 \qquad\qquad [6]$$
$$(0.10) \qquad\qquad (0.39)$$

$$n = 71 \quad s = 0.274 \quad r = 0.964$$

This seems to confirm the prediction for the activities of polysubstituted compounds made by Eq. 3 formulated from activities of "mono" substituted compounds. Most physicochemical parameter terms appearing in Eqs 3, 4 and 5 for substituent effects at each position are included in Eq. 6 as such, indicating that the substituent effects at various positions are almost additive in nature.

In Eq. 6, a $\Sigma\pi(6,7,8)$ term is used for the analysis. Correlations of only slightly poorer quality were in fact observed by using either $\pi(7)$ or log P instead of $\Sigma\pi(6,7,8)$. This is due to the fact, that the range of variations in π value for R^7 substituents (5.2) is much broader than those for R^1 (2.5), R^6 (1.7) and R^8 (1.0) substituents. The variations in $\Sigma\pi(6,7,8)$ and log P are mainly determined by that in $\pi(7)$, and the collinearity (r) of $\pi(7)$ with $\Sigma\pi(6,7,8)$ and log P is 0.94 and 0.92, respectively, for 71 compounds. Thus, even though the hydrophobicity is significant only for the R^7 substituents when analysed separately, the hydrophobicity of the whole molecule seems to play an important role, possibly in the transport process to the active site. Due to a joint effect of substituents, the $\Sigma F(6,7,8)$ term becomes significant in Eq. 6 indicating that an electron-donating effect on the 4-oxo function from the homocyclic moiety favours the activity through an electronic interaction with certain receptor sites. In this respect, inductive electron-

withdrawing substituents such as Cl at the 8-position are rather unfavourable to the activity.

With this information, and after considering the actual antibacterial
effects against infections due to various bacteria, as well as the toxicity
and the cost of synthesis, they selected AM-715 (5) as the objective
compound [$\log(1/\text{m.i.c.}) = 6.6$]. This compound shows much more

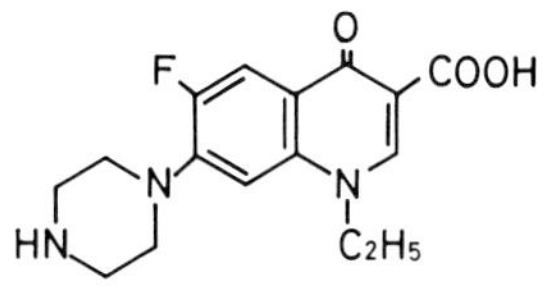

5

potent antibacterial activity (16- to 500-fold that of nalidixic acid
depending upon the bacterial species) and a much broader antibacterial
spectrum than any analogues previously developed. Especially striking
is the effect against Gram-negative bacteria, including that against
Pseudomonas, which is more potent than that of gentamicin. At present,
extensive clinical trials are being performed in a number of countries.
In Italy it has been marketed by Merck quite recently. The most active
compound included in Eq. 6 is a tricyclic 6,7,8-trisubstituted derivative
(6), $\log(1/\text{m.i.c.}) = 7.2$, which seems to possess an ideally optimized
structure in every respect suggested by the correlation.

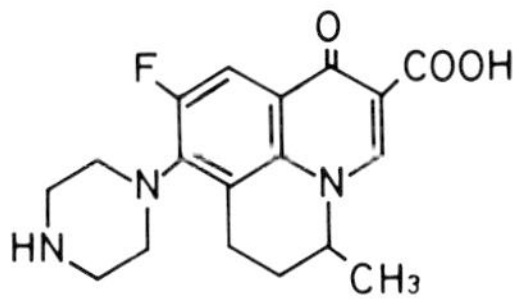

6

Design of a Novel *N*-Benzylacylamide Herbicide, S-47

In recent years, such perennials as bulrush (*Scirpus juncoides*) and
arrowhead (*Sagittaria pygmaea*) are the most serious pest weeds in
paddy fields in Japan (Ueki, 1983). Since they grow with perennial
stumps and tubers located under a certain depth of soil, they are difficult to eradicate by applying conventional herbicides only to the part
of the weeds above ground.

Quite recently, Kirino and his co-workers of Sumitomo Chemical
Company, Osaka, have developed a novel broad spectrum herbicide,

$$\langle\text{ring}\rangle \begin{array}{ccc} CH_3 & O & CH_3 \\ | & || & | \\ -C-NHCCH-C-CH_3 \\ | & | & | \\ CH_3 & Br & CH_3 \end{array}$$

7

S-47 (7), which is effective not only against annual but also against perennial weeds (Kamoshita and Kirino, 1982; Kirino *et al.*, 1981). In the course of the development, indications and predictions derived from QSAR analyses for related pesticides were successfully utilized, along with those for its own congeneric series of compounds.

These authors previously found that *N*-substituted aminoacetonitriles (8) exhibit remarkable effects in preventing soil-borne plant diseases,

$$R-NHCH_2CN$$

8

especially those due to *Fusarium* (Kirino *et al.*, 1980a). They determined the preventive effect against "yellows" of the Japanese radish, a disease caused by *Fusarium oxysporum*, in terms of the 50% preventive dose, ED_{50}(mole), applied to a certain volume of soil where the radish is grown. Equation 7 was formulated for 16 compounds where R is varied from *n*-alkyl (Me, Pr, Bu, Hex, etc.) to branched substituents (*i*-Pr, *t*-Bu, neoPent, 2,3-Me$_2$-2-Bu, etc.) as well as to cycloalkyls (*cyc*-Pr, -Hex, -Hept, etc.) (Kirino *et al.*, 1980b).

$$\log(1/ED_{50}) = 0.606E_s^c + 1.518 \qquad [7]$$
$$(0.184) \qquad (0.265)$$

$$n = 16 \quad s = 0.204 \quad r = 0.884$$

E_s^c is the Hancock "corrected" steric constant which is taken to be a parameter emphasizing the effect of branching, in addition to steric bulk (Fujita and Iwamura, 1983). The collinearity between E_s^c and π being insignificant (r = −0.53), Eq. 7 shows that the bulkier and the more branched the *N*-substituents, the higher is the activity. Since the activity determination requires a period of a few weeks using seedlings grown on the soil infected with the fungi, a part of the applied dose may be degraded during the test period. The Sumitomo workers considered that the steric bulk of *N*-substituents has a role in protecting the compounds against degradation, and that the stability is the critical factor determining the activity (Kirino *et al.*, 1980b).

Fujinami and his co-workers, including the present author, found another example in which the steric bulk of substituents enhances the herbicidal activity against annual grass weeds (Fujinami *et al.*, 1976). For the activity against a barnyard grass, *Echinochloa crus-galli* var. *frumentaceus*, of a series of *N*-chloroacetyl-*N*-phenylglycine ethyl esters having various substituents at the *ortho-* and *meta*-positions (9): X = *o*- and/or *m*-alkyl, -alkoxy, -halo, -acyl, -NO$_2$, -CF$_3$ and -Ph), they derived Eq. 8,

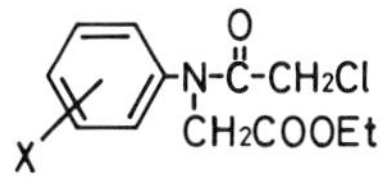

9

$$pI_{50} = -0.767E_s^{ortho} - 0.218E_s^{meta} + 3.990 \qquad [8]$$
$$\phantom{pI_{50} = } (0.158) \qquad (0.196) \qquad (0.240)$$

$$n = 28 \quad s = 0.295 \quad r = 0.905$$

where I$_{50}$ is the molar concentration of the solution (in a laboratory test) required to inhibit the shoot elongation to half the length of the control (Fujinami *et al.*, 1976).

This class of chloroacetamide herbicides, such as allidochlor (10) and butachlor (11), have been considered to exert their activity by

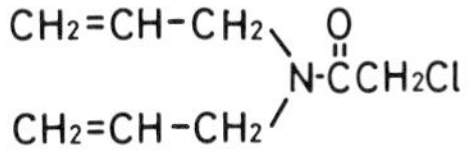

10

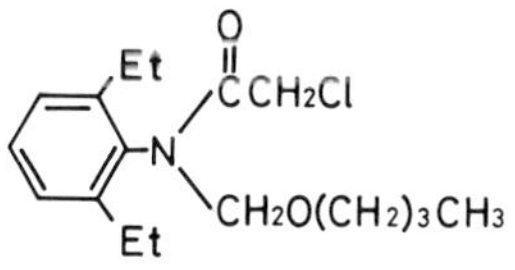

11

alkylation of the SH groups of certain proteases in the plant (Jaworski, 1975). Electron-attracting *N*-substituents are thought to be favourable to this type of activity and their steric bulk, if large, is considered to prevent the proper fit with the target. Contrary to expectation, however, Eq. 8 shows that the activity is not related to an electronic effect, but is potentiated by an increase in the steric bulkiness of the *ortho* and *meta* substituents. This result was attributed to an inhibition of interaction with some detoxication enzyme. They considered that the stability in the plant plays a decisive role in governing the potency (Fujinami *et al.*, 1976).

Kirino and co-workers applied the above conclusions relating the stability to pesticidal activity to the structural optimization of a series of newly discovered herbicide congeners, the N-benzylacylamides (12) which have an amide moiety in common with the N-chloroacetyl

12

phenylglycine esters (9) (Kamoshita and Kirino, 1982). Systematic modification of the structure was carried out to make the substituent R in (12) more and more bulky to increase the protection against the possible hydrolytic detoxication mechanism.

The analysis for a set of 41 derivatives, in which R varies from simple normal and branched alkyls (Me, Et, Pr, Hept, Oct, cyc-Pr, t-Bu, t-BuCH$_2$, i-BuCH$_2$, cyc-Hex, cyc-HexCH$_2$, etc.) to such congested groups as t-Bu(Cl)CH, t-Bu(Br)CH, i-Pr(Me)$_2$C and Me$_2$BrCBrCH, gave Eq. 9 (Kirino et al., 1982),

$$pI_{50} = -0.151\,\pi^2 + 0.983\,\pi - 0.350E_s^c + 2.877 \qquad [9]$$
$$\phantom{pI_{50} = }(0.093) \qquad (0.457) \qquad (0.070) \qquad (0.465)$$

$$n = 41 \quad s = 0.267 \quad r = 0.933$$

where I$_{50}$ is the molar concentration of the test solution required for 50% inhibition of shoot elongation of the seedlings of the bulrush. In Eq. 9, compounds where R = CH$_2$Br and CH$_2$Cl are not included, since their pI$_{50}$ values are about 1.5 units higher than those predicted by Eq. 9. This was attributed to higher reactivity of their halogens, probably in an alkylation reaction. These groups having primary halogen, however, are not favourable as a structural feature, since the E$_s^c$ value is made less negative, and the π value is not modified greatly. For haloalkyl groups where the halogen atom is not primary, the reactivity of the halogen seems to be reduced. The pI$_{50}$ values of these compounds fit Eq. 9 quite well, as do those of compounds without haloalkyl groups. This suggests that the activity of this series of compounds is not due to their alkylating properties, even though they have α-halogenoacyl substituents. Substituents R having a double bond at the α,β-position, and those having a β-halogen which could give an α,β-double bond by an elimination reaction, were also deleted from Eq. 9. Since conjugation with the carbonyl function may perturb the reactivity of the amide moiety, the actual activities are about 0.5 log unit lower than the values predicted by Eq. 9.

Equation 9 indicates that, although there is an optimum in hydrophobicity within the set of 41 compounds ($\pi_{opt} = 3.3$), the steric bulkiness of the R substituent in terms of E_s^c still needs to be augmented to obtain higher activity. Further structural modifications were made on the α-bromoacylamide structure (13). For 14 derivatives where R′ is

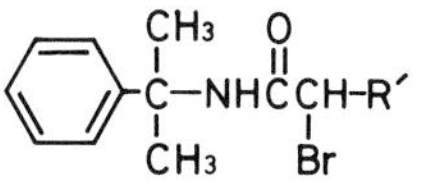

13

varied from a simple alkyl to such highly branched groups as i-$Pr(Me)_2C$, i-$Bu(Me)_2C$, and $(Et)_2MeC$, Eq. 10 was derived to show that the optimum for the steric bulk of R′ lies at about -3.1 in terms of E_s^c (Kirino, 1982).

$$pI_{50} = -0.199(E_s^c)^2 - 1.227E_s^c + 4.393 \qquad [10]$$
$$\quad\quad (0.152) \quad\quad\quad (0.546) \quad\quad (0.364)$$

$$n = 14 \quad s = 0.242 \quad r = 0.940$$

The E_s^c value for R′ is used in Eq. 10, since the value for such highly congested groups as R′CHBr cannot be estimated with sufficient accuracy.

Equation 10 indicates that the R substituent should not be made infinitely bulkier. Beyond the optimum, the fit with its own receptor could be inhibited. In this respect, it should be noted that the steric bulk of the second largest subgroup R^2 of the R substituents [$R = R^1R^2R^3C$; $F_s^c(R^1) > F_s^c(R^2) > F_s^c(R^3)$] has a specific effect on the activity (Kirino, 1982). When the R substituent is such that the R^2 subgroup is bulkier than Et, the activity is always considerably lower (by $0.7 - 1.4$ log units) than that estimated by means of Eq. 9 using the normal $E_s^c(R)$ value. These derivatives also are not used in deriving Eq. 9. Even though the steric bulk is below the optimum, too great a congestion of the acyl moiety would be deleterious to their fit with their own receptor.

Although the details are not shown here, quantitative analyses of the effect of substituents in the benzylamine moiety confirmed that the α,α'-dimethyl substitution and lack of aromatic substitution are optimal for high activity (Kirino, 1982).

Using this information and taking into consideration a certain (but not too serious) collinearity between E_s^c and π values for the compounds included in Eq. 10, as well as their ease of preparation, S-47 (13; R′ = t-Bu), where $\pi(R) = 2.2$ and $E_s^c(R') = -2.5$, was selected as a promising novel paddy field herbicide and taken forward to extensive field trials and toxicity tests (Kirino *et al.*, 1981). The activity of this compound, determined by the laboratory test against the bulrush shoot growth, is about 100 times that of the chloroacetyl lead compound. The α,α'-dimethyl substitution also enhances the activity about ten fold.

The field trials showed that S-47 in fact controls various weeds in paddy fields such as *Echinochloa crus-galli, Monochoria vaginalis, Cyperus serotinus, Eleocharis acicularis, Eleocharis kuroguwai* and *Sagittaria pygmaea*, in addition to the bulrush, *Scirpus juncoides*. Especially sensitive is the bulrush, which is killed at rates of 100–500 g/ha with complete safety to the rice plant (Kirino *et al.*, 1981). The broad herbicidal spectrum has been shown to be due not only to its intrinsic activity, but also to its moderate degrees of persistency and its mobility in soil (Kirino *et al.*, 1982). It is expected to be marketed soon in Japan, South Korea and Taiwan.

Conclusion

The above are among the most successful examples of quantitative drug design research in the generation of new drugs of practical use in Japan. The Hansch approach was skilfully used in these examples to optimize the lead structure, by aiming at "better" compounds predicted by correlation equations. The procedure was such that the prediction was made in the first example by assuming that the substituent effects at various positions in a molecule are additive. In the second example, transposition and extrapolation of quantitative information relating to the substituent effects led to the optimum structure. In each case, the potency was enhanced to more than 100 times that of the lead compound. Without the quantitative procedure, predictions and optimizations could only have been achieved with much greater difficulty. These examples might be considered as representing only a few cases among many other unsuccessful trials. Nevertheless, the fact that the successful examples have been consecutively accumulated recently is a great encouragement to our efforts to further elaborate QSAR methodology.

Acknowledgements

The author expresses his sincere thanks to the Organizing Committee of the Rhône-Poulenc Round Table Conference for inviting him to present this paper. He is also very grateful to Drs Hiroshi Koga and Osamu Kirino for permission to use their unpublished results. Those who wish to learn of their QSAR research in more detail are kindly asked to write to them directly at the following addresses: Hiroshi Koga (present address) New Drug Research Laboratories, Chugai Pharmaceutical Company, 3–41–8 Takada, Toshimaku, Tokyo 171, Japan. Osamu Kirino, Research Department, Pesticide Division, Sumitomo Chemical Company, 4–2–1 Takatsukasa, Takarazuka, Hyogo 665, Japan.

References

Albrecht, R. (1977). *Fortschr. Arzneimittelforsch.* **21**, 9–104.

Cramer, R.D., Snader, K.M., Willis, C.R., Chakrin, L.W., Thomas, J. and Sutton, B.M. (1979). *J. Med. Chem.* **22**, 714–725.

Fujinami, A., Satomi, T., Mine, A. und Fujita, T. (1976). *Pestic. Biochem. Physiol.* **6**, 287–295.

Fujita, T. (1978). "Structure–Activity Relationships – Quantitative Approaches: Significance in Drug Design and Mode-of-Action Studies". Nankodo, Tokyo.

Fujita, T. (1982). "Structure–Activity Relationships – Quantitative Approaches: Applications to Drug Design and Mode-of-Action Studies". Nankodo, Tokyo.

Fujita, T. and Iwamura, H. (1983). *In* "Steric Effects in Drug Design" (I. Motoc and M. Charton, eds), pp. 119–157. Springer Verlag, Berlin.

Hansch, C. and Fujita, T. (1964). *J. Am. Chem. Soc.* **86**, 1616–1626.

Hansch, C. (1976). *J. Med. Chem.* **19**, 1–6.

Hansch, C. and Leo, A. (1979). "Substituent Constants for Correlation Analysis in Chemistry and Biology". John Wiley & Sons, New York.

Jaworski, E.G. (1975). *In* "Herbicides: Chemistry, Degradation and Mode of Action Vol. 1" (P.C. Kearney and D.D. Kaufman, eds), pp. 349–376. Marcel Dekker Inc., New York.

Kamoshita, K. and Kirino, O. (1982). *In* "Structure–Activity Relationships – Quantitative Approaches: Applications to Drug Design and Mode-of-Action Studies" (T. Fujita, ed.), pp. 203–227. Nankodo, Tokyo.

Kirino, O., Oshita, H., Oishi, T. and Kato, T. (1980a). *Agric. Biol. Chem.* **44**, 25–30.

Kirino, O., Oshita, H., Oishi, T. and Kato, T. (1980b). *Agric. Biol. Chem.* **44**, 31–34.

Kirino, O., Furuzawa, K., Matsumoto, H., Hino, N. and Mine, A. (1981). *Agric. Biol. Chem.* **45**, 2669–2670.

Kirino, O., Furuzawa, K., Takayama, C., Matsumoto, H. and Mine, A. (1982). *In* "Abstracts of Papers presented at 5th International Congress of Pesticide Chemistry, Kyoto, 1982", IId–15.

Kirino, O. (1982). Personal communication.

Koga, H., Itoh, A., Murayama, S., Suzue, S. and Irikura, T. (1980). *J. Med. Chem.* **23**, 1358–1363.

Koga, H. (1982). *In* "Structure–Activity Relationships – Quantitative Approaches: Applications to Drug Design and Mode-of-Action Studies" (T. Fujita, ed.), pp. 177–202.

Kutter, E. and Hansch, C. (1969). *J. Med. Chem.* **12**, 647–652.

Lesher, G.Y., Froelich, E.J., Gruett, M.D., Bailey, J.H. and Brundage, R.P. (1962). *J. Med. Pharm. Chem.* **5**, 1063–1065.

Martin, Y.C. (1981). *J. Med. Chem.* **24**, 229–237.

Minami, S. (1975). *In* "Drug Design" (S. Yamabe, ed.), pp. 145–162. Asakura Shoten, Tokyo.

Ueki, K. (1983). *In* "Pesticide Chemistry: Human Welfare and the Environment", Vol. 2 (J. Miyamoto, ed.), pp. 319–324. Pergamon Press, Oxford.

Unger, S.H. (1980). *Drug Design* **11**, 47–119.

Wooldridge, K.R.H. (1980). *In* "Drugs Affecting the Respiratory System" (D.L. Temple, ed.), pp. 117–123. American Chemical Society, Washington, D.C.

Discussion

Chairman: Professor Rabin

Dr Dearden
In connection with the antibacterial series, I would like to ask the reasoning behind the selection of the steric parameters used in the correlations. In some cases E_s was used and in others the Verloop parameters, L and B_4; all very different.

Professor Fujita
The investigators used standard physicochemical parameters such as E_s, MR and STERIMOL values, and selected the statistically best equation. This empirical approach was used because industrial scientists want to derive equations which can be used predictively to guide synthesis of further compounds, which in this case was successful.

Dr Wold
I would like to ask Professor Fujita his views on the assumption of the additivity of the substituent effects. In the first example for instance, is it valid to assume additivity if only one substituent position at a time is varied?

Professor Fujita
It is dangerous always to assume additivity. In the case of the first series, since the 6, 7, and 8 positions are adjacent, the additivity of substituent effects would not always have been the case. There is a possibility of interaction among substituents. However the correlations showed that additivity was the case in this example.

Dr Caton
With regard to the nalidixic acid analogues, Professor Fujita has shown that QSAR techniques were used to produce a more active antibacterial compound. But, at the same time, this compound also had a broader spectrum of antibacterial action. Did the QSAR help to predict this, or was it just an accidental finding?

Professor Fujita
I do not know whether or not it was an accidental finding. What the investigators wanted to do, however, was to use the Hansch technique to develop a novel compound. Perhaps they were lucky, in terms of finding a compound which was more potent as well as having a wider spectrum of activity.

Mr Depaire
In Professor Fujita's conclusions, he stated that the Hansch analysis is an extrapolation. But, from the slides, it seems to me that it is an interpolation.

Professor Fujita
In the second example, 41 compounds were first synthesized, and the correlation equation showed that the steric bulkiness needed to be increased for high activity — that means that they extrapolated the concept. Finally, they derived a parabolic equation, so at the final stage it might be interpolation.

Mr Depaire
Is it possible to estimate the increase in the number of compounds which need to be synthesized because of this extrapolation procedure?

Professor Fujita
They should have made a smaller number of compounds to use the quantitative procedure efficiently. However, the chemistry was so routine they tended to make more than the minimum number.

Professor Clementi
I am rather worried about the use of the squared terms together with the linear terms in multiple regression analysis. As far as I understood these are highly correlated, which might give rise to multi-collinearities in multiple regression analysis if only these two are used, and there might, therefore, be meaningless results.

Secondly, I do not understand the chemical significance of the squared term. Has Professor Fujita any comment to make on either of these two points?

Professor Fujita
Sometimes there is high collinearity between a linear and a squared parameter. However it is a very convenient way, in practical terms, to demonstrate an optimum value. I believe that an optimum does exist in these correlations as shown by the parabolic curve on the slides. I agree that it would be of interest to explore the physicochemical meaning in greater detail.

3 Computational Chemistry and Receptor Characterization

G.R. MARSHALL

Department of Physiology and Biophysics,
Washington University School of Medicine,
660 South Euclid Avenue, St. Louis, Missouri 63110, USA

Introduction

Through a discussion of our work on computer-aided drug design, I would hope to be convincing about two facts. First, computational chemistry has come of age. Because of the increasing availability of powerful computational hardware and of the advances in our basic understanding of theoretical chemistry, the chemist now has the possibility of calculating many properties of molecules which have not yet been synthesized, and of being reasonably assured that the synthetic molecule will, in fact, exhibit those properties. The second thing to be emphasized is that computer graphics is a very effective means of communicating between the chemist and his computations. One can view the computer as a multidimensional notebook to assist in the definition of hypotheses, to test hypotheses for consistency with known structure–activity data, and to help design novel compounds for synthesis and testing. Computers generate lots of numbers; numbers themselves do not mean much to chemists. One would like to distill the relevant information in a meaningful way and to communicate that experience. There are many levels of details that can be presented; space-filling models, stick figures, colour-coded surfaces and more creative displays to try and bridge the communication gap. The different methods, in

DRUG DESIGN: FACT OR FANTASY
ISBN 0.12.388180.3

terms of what is actually seen graphically, do much to add credibility to the computations. They provide a basis for the chemist to verify that what has been calculated may have some physical reality.

Strategy

In terms of drug design, the key feature is the shape of the molecule when it interacts with the receptor. Unfortunately, we generally lack detailed information about the receptor. All the physical tools that might be used, such as crystallography or NMR, deal in general with the conformation of the molecule in the absence of the receptor. We have thus chosen to test the concept of the pharmacophore, to see whether this idea can, in fact, be used to deduce the molecular shape when bound to the receptor. The basic idea is one which should be familiar, that is, there are several groups in a molecule which are more important than others. These are the groups which are the primary determinants of recognition, i.e. those groups essential to activity.

It is the three-dimensional arrangement of those groups which is critical for activation. In fact, the three-dimensional arrangement can be uniquely represented as a point in a multidimensional distance space that we call "orientation space". Thus, the triangle, AB, BC, AC, where AB is the distance between essential groups A and B, etc., can be represented as a single point in this space and represents a three-point pharmacophore hypothesis. If the concept of a pharmacophore is correct, it can be argued that, in terms of recognition, it does not really matter what composes the backbone as long as it does not compete with the receptor for occupancy. It is the groups A, B, C, ... N and their relative positions in space that are important. This says nothing about potency, but if we do not have the critical three-dimensional pattern we shall not have any activation at the receptor. Since the shape of the drug at the receptor is generally not known, one can only hypothesize the groups A, B, C, ... N which are important. One can then determine the conformational space allowed for the molecule of interest, letting the computer examine all possible conformations. For each allowed conformation, one can determine the pharmacophore, that is, triangle, in the case of A, B, and C, plotting that as a single point in orientation space. If that is done for a series of drugs, and if the idea of pharmacophore is correct, that is, each one of these molecules possesses a common pattern, it is possible to intersect the set of orientation maps, and find all the three-dimensional arrangements of groups which are pharmacophore candidates.

To summarize the strategy advocated, one first determines the sterically-allowed conformations, that is, examine all possible conformations of a drug, because it is not known what will be the effect of interaction with the receptor on selecting a particular conformer. One then transforms to an appropriate space – orientation space – and, as medicinal chemists, use the basic concept that some groups and some atoms are more important than others. In general, heteroatoms, lone pairs, pi-centres, planar groups, etc. are the "hot spots" for examination. Again, candidate pharmacophores are determined by their presence throughout the set of molecules which interact with a given receptor. Once a unique pattern is found exploitation begins.

Once one has a particular pharmacophore hypothesis, it improves the efficiency of the computational problem in looking at new molecules by determining whether they are capable of presenting that particular pharmacophore which certainly helps in the decision about what to make next. Mapping of the receptor – biophase interface is also possible; in other words, one can probe sterically where on the molecular framework new chemistry can be done.

Perhaps the most exciting possibility is the chance of controlling cross-reactivity. Side-effects are probably the major drawback to current therapeutics, anything that can be done to reduce side-effects is clearly an improvement. By building receptor files and by being more specific about requirements for particular activities, there is a chance of reducing side-effects. The clearer the picture we have of the lock, the more specific we can be in the design of a key.

Example – Neuroleptics

A common problem, obviously, is to identify the pharmacophore. Rigid compounds which bind to the dopamine receptor such as apomorphine, octoclothepin and butaclamol offer a good example because this is a case on which much of the methodology was developed. This problem was brought to our attention by Dr. Leslie Humber of Ayerst, who first synthesised the butaclamol series of neuroleptics. Apomorphine, which is an agonist at this receptor, has a cryptic dihydroxyphenethylamine, dopamine, within it. In collaboration with Dr. Humber (Humber *et al.*, 1975), we found that it was possible to make the one ring from each of the three rigid compounds coincident and coplanar, while allowing the nitrogens to occupy basically the same position in space. Based on this observation, it can be argued that the pharmacophore for this system is an aromatic ring and a nitrogen, in a specific distance from the ring, and a specific height above the plane of the ring.

That is a reasonable hypothesis, but how can it be checked? How can one make sure that there is some validity in the concept? First, one can look at other things that are known about the system. Apomorphine is stereospecific, i.e. the optical isomer has no activity at the receptor. But the hypothetical pharmacophore has a mirror plane of symmetry; it is a ring and a nitrogen. Certainly, therefore, the inactive isomer of apomorphine can also present the pharmacophore simply by reflection of the active compound (Fig. 1). Obviously, the fit to the pharmacophore for both is extremely good. The question is "Why does the optical

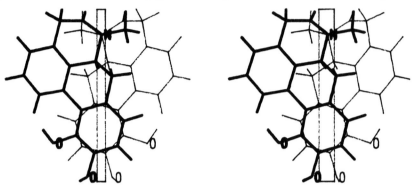

FIG. 1   Stereo view* of inactive isomer of apomorphine (dark lines) generated by reflection of apomorphine (light lines) through mirror plane containing ring centre and nitrogen.

isomer of apomorphine not bind to the receptor?" One possibility is competition with the receptor for volume occupancy. One can examine the combined volume map of compounds which do bind to the receptor to see whether the inactive isomer of apomorphine requires something novel. If it does, it can be postulated that it is competing with the receptor for some part of the novel volume, and thus, unable to present the activating pattern.

The computer has generated the volume of the inactive isomer of apomorphine, and subtracted all the volume required by a set of active compounds (about 10) which bind at this receptor, and which are conformationally restricted. Two novel areas of volume are required by the inactive isomer and not by any active compound examined to date. One could, therefore, argue that the receptor has some occupancy of these volumes, so that any new compound that we try to synthesize, which required the total novel area, would be predicted to be inactive. If it required only partial amounts of that area, it would not, of course, be possible to be so sure about its potential activity or inactivity.

A related problem presented itself during a lecture in Brussels at the

---

* A "stereo-viewer", suitable for use with Fig. 1, has been designed by Professor F. Vögtle and distributed by Verlag Chemie (obtainable from the Royal Society of Chemistry in England).

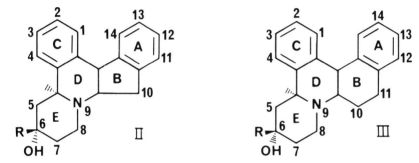

FIG. 2   Neuroleptic candidates based on butaclamol I R = *t*-butyl. II = exo-5 = 6-R-6-hydroxy-5,6,7,8,9,14b-hexahydro-4bH-indeno(2,3,-c)pyrido(1,2-a)isoquinoline.   III = exo-6 = 6-R-6-hydroxy-5,6,7,8,9,10,11,15b-octahydro-4bH-benzo(a)pyrido(1,2,-f) phenanthridine.

laboratory of Professor Van Binst. The two analogues, II and III, of butaclamol I shown in Fig. 2 had been synthesized (Laus *et al.*). The motivation for doing so was as follows: there are two possible conformers of the 7-membered ring system, depending upon the torsional rotation about the ethylene bridge between the two aromatic rings. While one of the conformers is seen in the crystal structure (conformer A), the other conformer (conformer B) is the one predicted to interact with the receptor because it puts the nitrogen and the ring in the right positions relative to apomorphine. Using energy calculations on butaclamol itself, the difference between conformer A and conformer B is about 0.5 kcal; it is "noise" level and crystal packing forces could easily select between the two. By modelling these two analogues with Dreiding models (Laus *et al.*), the exo-6-membered ring locks the compound in conformer A and the exo-5-membered ring analogue locks the compound in conformer B. Initial inspection of Dreiding models suggested that both would occupy part of the area required by the inactive isomer of apomorphine and would, therefore, be predicted to be inactive.

It is interesting to see what the computer has to say about this problem. Shown in Fig. 3 is the minimized structure of the 6-membered ring, compared with conformer B of butaclamol. The first thing that

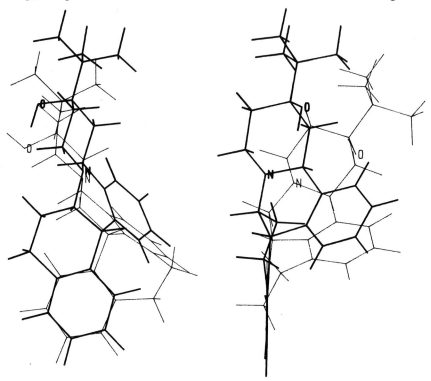

FIG. 3   Orthogonal views of exo-6 (dark lines) compared with conformer B of butaclamol (light lines).

is quite apparent is that there has been a large movement in the nitrogen position. In conformer A the nitrogen is much closer to the plane. Again, conformer A is not the active conformer; one thinks it is conformer B that is active. One could say, therefore, that the exo-6 analogue is probably inactive because it prefers conformer A by 6 kcal or more to conformer B.

The other big change, though, is the movement of the *t*-butyl and hydroxyl groups on position three. That is very important because in the butaclamol series these groups form an important accessory binding site. If the *t*-butyl and hydroxyl groups are removed, there is no activity (Humber *et al.*, 1979a), the analogue does not have sufficient affinity for the receptor. For the butaclamol series of neuroleptics, this functionality is a critical accessory binding site. In fact, if it is moved from the three position to the adjacent two position, all the activity is lost (Humber *et al.*, 1979b). The computer, in effect, states that the analogue (exo-6) has accommodated the substitution by forcing the *t*-butyl and hydroxyl groups to shift as well as moving the nitrogen. Both reasons would predict that the exo-6-analogue would be inactive.

Examination of the 5-membered ring system, in Fig. 4 shows a good preservation of conformer B, i.e. the nitrogen is approximately in the same relative position, But again, the *t*-butyl-hydroxyl group has

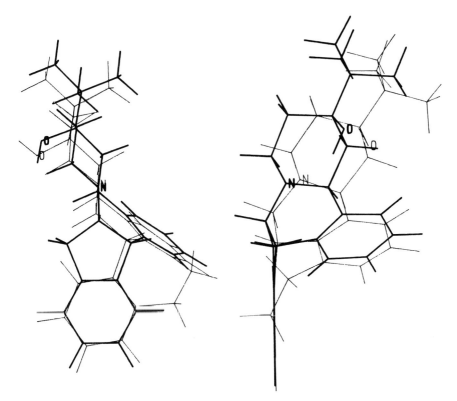

FIG. 4   Orthogonal views of exo-5 (light lines) compared with conformer B of butaclamol (light lines).

moved. Humber has shown (Voith *et al.*, 1978) that increasing the bulk of the *t*-butyl group gave a sharp loss in activity. The exo-5 analogue moves the *t*-butyl-hydroxyl groups on position three towards the two position as occupied by butaclamol in which Humber has shown that substitution leads to an inactive analogue. Therefore, one would also predict this analogue to be inactive. Both compounds turn out to be essentially inactive (Laus *et al.*). On the one hand, it is unfortunate that this study is retrospective because of the synthetic effort expended; on the other, the compounds add additional information to the understanding of the butaclamol—receptor interaction.

This is the sort of symbiosis that arises from the computer and the chemist working together. The chemist can examine compounds which have not yet been prepared; he can make predictions based on what is known about other series; he can search conformational space to see whether his ideas about important groups and the pharmacophore are consistent across a series and so on. Then he can synthesize and test his compounds, and refine his hypothesis as necessary.

The Conformational Variable

There is another area which is also as important, that is the idea of considering the conformational variable as a parameter that one wants to monitor. In most cases, one is presented with molecules with a tremendous degree of flexibility. Modifications are often made without considering that those modifications could dramatically alter the possible shapes that the molecule can assume. One of the things that should be done routinely is to examine the conformational effects prior to synthesis. There are also modifications that one can make, as chemists, to change the conformational parameters: increasing steric bulk, introduction of ring constraints, introduction of unsaturation, etc.

A problem that occurs in peptide chemistry is the elimination of peptide bonds because they are labile to enzymatic hydrolysis. To achieve oral activity of peptides, much work has been done on the chemistry of dipeptide surrogates by substitutions that prevent enzymatic digestion (such as alpha-methyl groups, isosteric replacements of amide bonds, and so on). A great deal of work has gone, and is going, into this sort of chemistry. However, there is a problem in that many people do not examine the consequence of substitution before synthesis. One wants to make the amide bond resistant to hydrolysis, but one also wants to preserve the shape which interacts with the receptor. It is quite plausible that a good modification for giving stability to hydrolysis may, in fact, prevent the conformation that would interact with the receptor. One must find a way to assess that problem, i.e. can the appropriate conformations be mimicked by the analogue?

Assume that the *trans*-amide bond will be modified in the dipeptide surrogate, replacing the central amide bond of acetyl—alanyl—alanyl-methylamide with other groups. The *N*-terminal acetyl part will be common to all the analogues and serves as the frame of reference. Is it possible to point the side chain of the second residue, the alpha—beta bond vector in the same direction for the analogue as can be done for the parent amide? This would provide a means for assessing shape similarity. Unfortunately, it is unknown which direction is important because the conformation is not known which binds to the receptor. The problem, therefore, has to be approached statistically. For the parent compound, one records all the possible directions in which the alpha–beta vector can point, with respect to the *N*-acetyl frame, while examining the six major degrees of freedom which affect the relative position of the two vectors as shown in Fig. 5. This process of searching conformational space is then repeated for the analogue, looking for overlap of alpha–beta vectors with the parent.

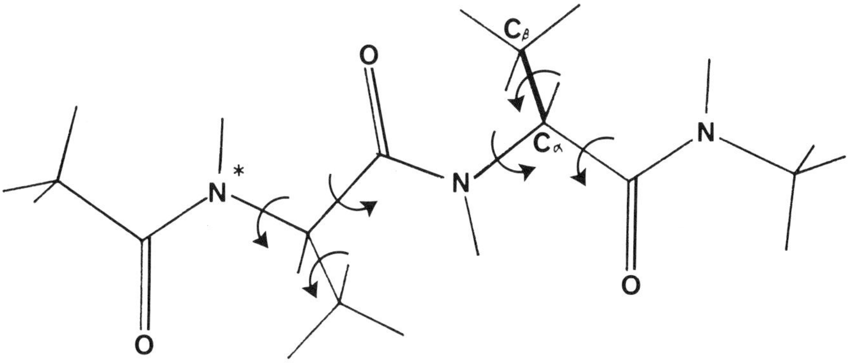

Angle increments: backbone 30° (0–330); side chains 30° (0–90).
Accuracy factor: 0.4 Å.

FIG. 5   Vector map search for trans amide control for peptide bond modification. Central amide bond is varied and carbon–alpha to carbon–beta vector recorded for each sterically allowed conformation.

Quite a number of possible amide-bond surrogates have been investigated. From 14 756 allowed conformers for the dipeptide, 186 unique alpha–beta vectors were obtained for the amide bond control. For the retro-amide, which has been advocated (Goodman *et al.*, 1979) as a good means of conferring resistance to hydrolysis, and which has approximately the same number of conformations (14080) as the normal peptide, an overlap of only 8% was found. The cases in which the retro-amide have been substituted have been singularly unimpressive. Most cases in which activity was retained are substituted into portions of peptides that do not affect activity (Marshall, 1982).

There are other candidates such as trans-double bonds with 66% overlap. That has been used effectively in enkephalin (Hann *et al.*, 1982, Cox *et al.*, 1980) in a position that matters. There are other successful surrogates: a ketomethylene group which has been used in an angiotensin converting enzyme (ACE) inhibitor (Almquist *et al.*, 1980), shows 97% overlap and the reduced amide with 100% overlap which has been used in a renin inhibitor (Szelke *et al.*, 1982).

These are not comparisons that can be done easily by chemical intuition. Consider the thioamide as a replacement. Because the sulphur atom is so much larger than oxygen, one might dismiss it. It turns out, however, that the bond length difference almost compensates for the size increase. Based on conformational analysis, the thioamide is a good mimic (56% overlap) of the amide bond itself.

Also of interest were *cis*-amide modifications. In fact, we had prepared the tetrazole analogue of the amide bond between residues two and three in TRH generating a molecule which was biologically inactive (Marshall, 1982). We did not know whether it was inactive because it could not assume the right conformation, or whether the carbonyl oxygen replaced might be involved in a hydrogen bond with the bulk of the tetrazole preventing the interaction. Overlap of only 23% between the tetrazole and the cis-amide suggests that either the trans-amide is required for activity in TRH, or that the tetrazole ring precludes the correct interaction with the receptor. We are in the process of preparing the trans- and cis-double bond substitution to investigate this problem further.

Conclusion

Molecular modelling has become a useful adjunct to the practising medicinal chemist. It allows the calculation of properties of molecules prior to their synthesis, the determination of the consistency of the chemist's current hypothesis with known structure–activity data, and a tenuous outline of the spatial feature of the target, the receptor. One can now examine the conformational effects of proposed modification in order to optimise the probability of an active analogue, and determine the information content if activity results. As a minimum, computer-aided drug design is a vast improvement on traditional molecular modelling techniques in that it allows superposition of non-congeneric series, etc. Its most impressive feature, however, is its potential as a multidimensional notebook to assist the individual chemist in the creative development of more specific therapeutic agents.

References

Almquist, R.G., Chao, R.R., Ellis, M.E. and Johnson, H.L. (1980). *J. Med. Chem.* **23**, 1392–1398.

Cox, M.T., Gorley, J.J., Hayward, C.F. and Petter, N.N. (1980). *J. Chem. Soc. Chem. Commun.*, 800–802.

Goodman, M. and Chorev, M. (1979). *Acc. Chem. Res.* **12**, 1–7.

Hann, M.M., Sammes, P.G., Kennewell, P.D. and Taylor, J.B. (1982). *J. Chem. Soc. Perkin Trans. I*, 307–314.

Humber, L.G., Bruderlein, F.T. and Voith, K. (1975). *Mol. Pharmacol.* **11**, 833–840.

Humber, L.G., Bruderlein, F.T., Philipp, A.H., Gotz, M. and Voith, K. (1979a). *J. Med. Chem.* **22**, 761–767.

Humber, L.G., Philipp, A.H., Bruderlein, F.T., Gotz, M. and Voith, K. (1979b). *In* "Computer-Assisted Drug Design" (E.C. Olson and R.E. Christoffersen, eds), pp. 227–241, ACS Symposium Series 112, Washington, D.C.

Laus, G. and Van Binst, G. Personal Communication.

Marshall, G.R. (1982). *In* "Chemical Regulation of Biological Mechanisms" (A.M. Greighton and S. Turner, eds), pp. 279–293, Chemical Society, London.

Szelke, M., Leckie, B., Hallett, A., Jones, D.M., Suieras, J., Atrash, B. and Lever, A.F. (1982). *Nature (London)* **299**, 555–557.

Voith, K., Bruderlein, F.T. and Humber, L.G. (1978). *J. Med. Chem.* **21**, 694–698.

Discussion

Chairman: Professor Rabin

Dr Palfreyman

You said that one of the future objectives of this work was perhaps to try to identify toxic centres in molecules. With regard to the dopamine compounds, has any work been done in this area, trying to find in the pharmacophore which part of it is giving rise to toxic effects? For example, in apomorphine, one of the medicinal chemist's greatest problems is the toxic nature of these compounds.

Professor Marshall

Dopamine pharmacology is so mobile that it is hard for the analysis to keep up with pharmacologists. That is one of the problems. All the data in the literature were collected pre-D1, D2, D3 and so on receptors, which makes some difficulty in the interpretation of those sorts of results.

The first general statement is that as medicinal chemists we have been, in our opinion, paid to optimize the wrong "end of the horse". We win by generating active compounds. If we look at a large data base of compounds generated by medicinal chemists and ask what percentage of compounds contain a cryptic phenethylamine, the answer is about 65–70%. If we then ask whether those compounds are rigid or flexible, we find that 95% of them are very flexible compounds. That tells me that the medicinal chemist responds to his environment. If he has a series of tests, and he is designing compounds, he will make compounds that will be active in one test or in another – but perhaps not the test on which he is supposedly working. Rigidity, because it is specific about the receptor we are trying to hit, is the way to overcome some of the side-effect problems.

Secondly, most of our methods have provided no insight into what the receptor is looking for. Therefore, we had to stay on the same active framework, usually associated with a large number of side-effects. I think that in being able to cross congeneric series we have the potential for solving some of these problems.

Professor Rabin

You will face formidable competition from the protein chemists because presumably it will be possible to do X-ray crystallography on the actual receptors.

Professor Marshall

I have no problem with accepting data from wherever it comes. There is nothing that I would rather see than an X-ray picture of the acetylcholine or the dopamine receptor. We have taken this approach because it is felt to be more representative of what is faced by the medicinal chemists.

Professor Rabin

The possibility of conformational changes in the receptor itself has not been taken into account. It is known for enzymes, such as carboxypeptidase, that there can be a movement of 12 Å of one group at the active site. Does this not create a problem which has not yet been tackled?

Professor Marshall

Every time we do NMR and IR spectra, it is clear that there is something going on in molecules in addition to the static images that even crystallographers present. Computational chemistry is coming of age; these things can be accommodated.

I regard what we are obtaining as not so much a physical picture of what an enzyme site looks like, but a functional representation, a functional framework to deal with structure – activity data.

4 Designing Prodrugs and Bioprecursors

C.G. WERMUTH

*Laboratoire de Chemie Organique, Faculté de
Pharmacie, Université Louis Pasteur, 74 Route du Rhin,
B.P. 10, 67048 Strasbourg Cedex, France*

Introduction

Therapeutic approaches based on molecular pharmacology mostly use *in vitro* models (membrane or enzyme preparations, cell or micro-organism cultures, isolated organs, etc.) In the last decade they gave rise to the discovery of numerous very potent and quite selective agents. As examples, we can mention the GABA-agonists muscimol and isoguvacine, the H_2 histamine antagonists burinamide and cimetidine, the dopaminergic agonists ADTN or peptides like the enkephalines or somatostatin.

However, the bioavailability of such molecules can be very unsatisfactory; as a matter of fact, due to their polarity, the functional groups which are present in the molecule may lead to poor absorption or to incorrect distribution. They may also, on account of their vulnerability, be the subject of an early metabolic destruction such as first-pass effects or any other kind of degradation leading to a short biological half-life. For these compounds the *in vivo* administration is limited to the parenteral route and their clinical usefulness is thus restricted. Sometimes an adequate pharmaceutical formulation (micro-encapsulation, sustained-release or enterosoluble preparations) can overcome these drawbacks but often the galenic formulation is inoperant and a chemical modification of the active molecule is necessary in order to correct its

DRUG DESIGN: FACT OR FANTASY
ISBN 0.12.388180.3

pharmacokinetic insufficiences. This chemical formulation process, whose objective is to convert an interesting active molecule into a clinically acceptable drug, involves very often the so-called "prodrug design".

Initially the term prodrug was introduced by Albert to describe "any compound which undergoes biotransformation prior to exhibiting its pharmacological effects" (Albert, 1958; Albert, 1964). Such a broad definition includes both accidental historic prodrugs (aspirin → salicylic acid) or active metabolites (imipramine → desmethylimipramine) and compounds intentionally prepared in order to improve the pharmacokinetic profile of an active molecule. From this point of view the term "drug latentiation" proposed by Harper (1959) is much more appropriate for prodrug design as it points out the intentional character of the approach. Drug latentiation is defined as "the chemical modification of a biologically active compound to form a new compound which, upon *in vivo* enzymatic attack, will liberate the parent compound". But even this definition is too broad and an attentive survey of the specialized literature led us to divide the prodrugs into two classes: the properly so-called prodrugs or carrier-linked prodrugs, and the bioprecursors (Wermuth, 1983).

The *carrier-linked prodrugs* result from a temporary linkage of the active molecule with a transport moiety which is mostly of lipophilic nature. A simple hydrolytic reaction cleaves this transport moiety at the adequate moment (e.g. bacampicillin, progabide). Such prodrugs are *per se* less active than the parent compounds or even inactive. The transport moiety (carrier group) will be chosen for its non toxicity and its ability to ensure the release of the active principle with efficient kinetics.

The *bioprecursors* do not imply a temporary linkage between the active principle and a carrier group, but result from a molecular modification of the active principle itself. This modification generates a new compound, able to be a substrate for the metabolizing enzymes, the metabolite being the expected active principle. This approach exemplifies the active metabolite concept in the previsional way (sulindac, fenbufen).

Carrier-Linked Prodrugs (Carrier Prodrugs)

The Prodrug Principle

The prodrug principle (Fig. 1) consists of "the attachment of a carrier group to the active drug to alter its physicochemical properties and then the subsequent enzyme attack to release the active drug moiety"

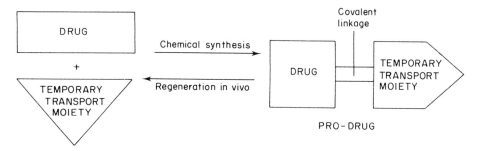

FIG. 1   The prodrug principle (Wermuth, 1981)

(Harper, 1959). "Prodrugs can thus be viewed as drugs containing specialized non-toxic protective groups utilized in a transient manner to alter or eliminate undesirable properties in the parent molecule" (Sinkula, 1977).

A well designed prodrug satisfies the following criteria (Higuchi *et al.*, 1975; Wermuth, 1978a; Wermuth, 1980a):

1) The linkage between the drug substance and the transport moiety is usually a covalent bond.

2) As a rule the prodrug is inactive or less active than the parent compound.

3) The linkage between the parent compound and the transport moiety must be broken *in vivo*.

4) The prodrug, as well as the *in vivo* released transport moiety, must be non toxic.

5) The generation of the active form must take place with rapid kinetics to ensure effective drug levels at the site of action and to minimize either direct prodrug metabolisation or gradual drug inactivation.

An example of prodrug design taking into account these criteria is found in orally active ampicillin derivatives (von Daehne *et al.*, 1970; Bodin *et al.*, 1975).

Ampicillin is one of the main representatives of the β-lactam antibiotics. This drug is widely used as a broad spectrum antibiotic, but it suffers from a poor absorption when administered orally; only about 40% of the drug is absorbed after oral administration. In other words, to achieve the same clinical efficiency and the same blood level, one must give two to three times more ampicillin by mouth than by intramuscular injection. The clinical tolerance of orally given ampicillin may be affected, the non-absorbed part of the drug destroying the intestinal flora. Therefore, numerous attempts have been made to improve these poor absorption properties.

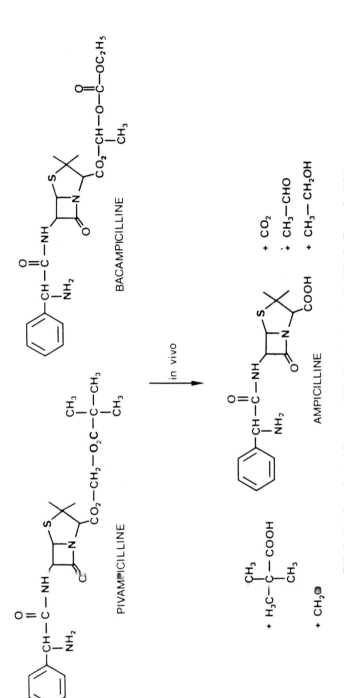

FIG. 2   Prodrugs derived from ampicillin (Von Daehne et al., 1970; Bodin et al., 1975)

Figure 2 represents two current prodrugs of ampicillin: pivampicillin and bacampicillin. Both result from the esterification of the polar carboxylic group with a lipophilic, enzymatically labile ester. The main properties of these two prodrugs can be summarised as follows:

1) The absorption of these compounds is nearly quantitative (98–99%).
2) The generation of free ampicillin in the blood stream is rapid (less than 15 minutes).
3) The released carrier molecules are formaldehyde and pivalic acid (trimethyl acetic acid) for pivampicillin and acetaldehyde, ethanol and carbon dioxide in the case of bacampicillin. These three latter compounds are natural metabolites in the human body. This may explain the better tolerance of bacampicillin compared with pivampicillin.
4) The serum levels attained following oral administration of bacampicillin are similar to those obtained after intramuscular injection of an equimolecular amount of free ampicillin.
5) The clinical trials confirm the efficiency and the safety of bacampicillin. Due to its good absorption, the drug is given at lower dosage than ampicillin: 0.8 g daily is sufficient in common infections as compared to 2.0 g daily for ampicillin.
6) It has been shown, and this seems to be a general rule fǒr prodrugs, that pivampicillin and bacampicillin are inactive *per se*, the antibiotic potency appearing only *in vivo* after the release of free ampicillin.

Practical Applications of Prodrug Design

The domain of application of the prodrug approach is illustrated in Fig. 3. In practice, carrier prodrugs achieve usually one of the four following goals: increased lipophilicity, water solubility, selective delivery, suppression of an undesirable organoleptic or physicochemical property ("chemical formulation").

Lipophilic carrier prodrugs
The attachment of a lipophilic carrier group to an active principle provides a better bioavailability, mostly by facilitating cell membrane crossing by passive diffusion.

Starting from hydroxylic derivatives high lipophilicity can simply be obtained by esterification (or sometimes etherification). Dipivaloylepinephrine for example (Fig. 4) crosses the cornea and is used in the treatment of glaucoma (McClure, 1975). In a similar manner, dibenzoyl-2-amino-6,7-dihydroxy-tetrahydronaphthalene (DB-ADTN) reaches the CNS, whereas the parent dopamine agonist ADTN does not (Horn, 1980). In the oestradiol prodrug oestradiol 3-benzoate 17-cyclooctenyl ether (EBCO), the phenolic hydroxyl group is masked as a benzoyl ester

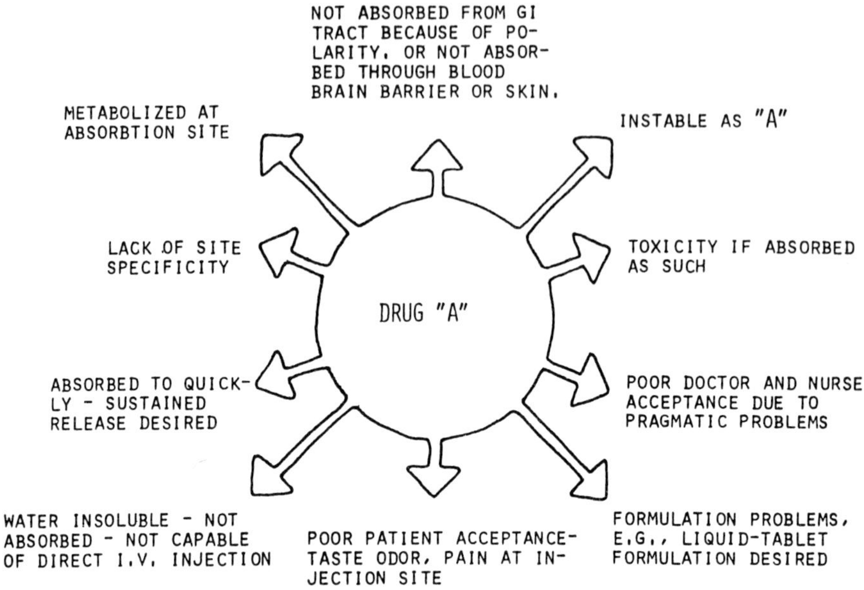

NOT ABSORBED FROM GI
TRACT BECAUSE OF PO-
LARITY, OR NOT ABSOR-
BED THROUGH BLOOD
BRAIN BARRIER OR SKIN,

METABOLIZED AT
ABSORBTION SITE

INSTABLE AS "A"

LACK OF SITE
SPECIFICITY

DRUG "A"

TOXICITY IF ABSORBED
AS SUCH

ABSORBED TO QUICK-
LY - SUSTAINED
RELEASE DESIRED

POOR DOCTOR AND NURSE
ACCEPTANCE DUE TO
PRAGMATIC PROBLEMS

WATER INSOLUBLE - NOT
ABSORBED - NOT CAPABLE
OF DIRECT I.V. INJECTION

POOR PATIENT ACCEPTANCE-
TASTE ODOR, PAIN AT IN-
JECTION SITE

FORMULATION PROBLEMS,
E.G., LIQUID-TABLET
FORMULATION DESIRED

Fig. 3   Shortcomings which may be overcome through chemical formulation (Higuchi and Stella, 1975; Wermuth, 1981)

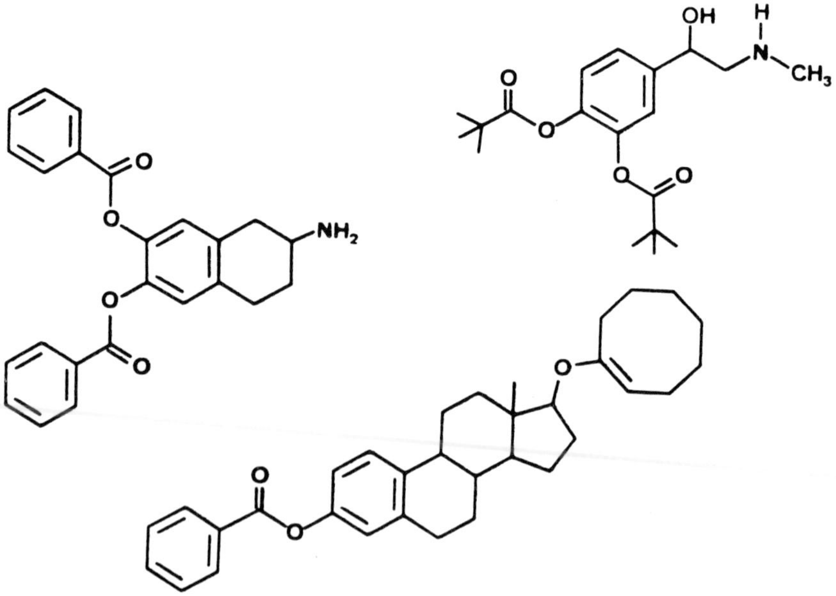

FIG. 4   Lipophilic derivatives of hydroxy compounds (McClure, 1975; Horn, 1980; Falconi *et al.*, 1972)

and the alcoholic 17-γ-hydroxyl, as an enol ether derived from cyclo-octanone. This derivative was designed for a sustained release formulation of oestradiol (Falconi *et al.*, 1972).

Lipophilic prodrugs can also be derived from a carboxylic function, the most commonly used derivatives being carboxylic esters. One can use simple esters of aliphatic alcohols, like tyrosine methyl ester (Anden *et al.*, 1966), nipecotic acid ethyl ester (Frey *et al.*, 1979) and γ-amino-butyric acid cetyl ester (Tsibina *et al.*, 1974; Ostrovskaya *et al.*, 1972), or lipoidal prodrugs in which the carboxyl function esterifies the free alcoholic hydroxyl of 1,2- or 1,3-diglyceride. Applied to the anti-inflammatory agent naproxen, this approach yielded the 2-esters of 1,3-dipalmitoylglycerol (Fig. 5) which gave less gastric irritation and higher plasma levels than the parent compound (Jones, 1980). The rationale for the design of lipoidal prodrugs is based on the well established principles concerning the intestinal absorption of natural triglycerides (Jones, 1980; Akesson *et al.*, 1978).

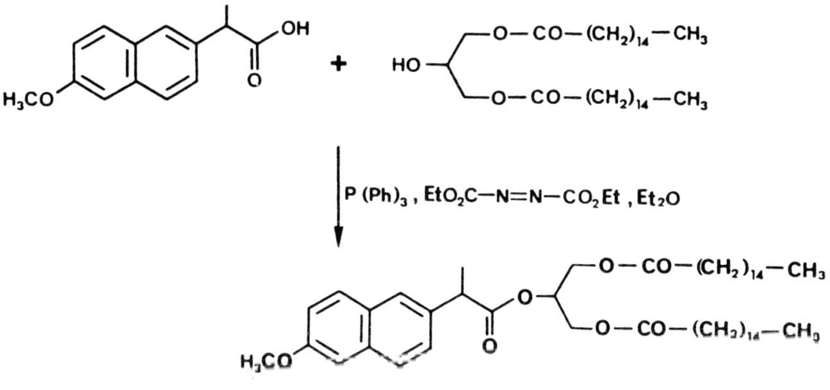

FIG. 5   Synthesis of the naproxen-2-glyceride (Jones, 1980)

The wide-spread use of acyloxymethyl esters in the antibiotic chemistry, as illustrated above for bacampicillin, was initiated by Jansen and Russel (1965) at Wyeth Laboratories and successfully applied to pivampicillin (von Daehne *et al.*, 1970), talampicillin (Clayton *et al.*, 1976) and also cephalosporins (Binderup *et al.*, 1971). In each of these cases, the oral absorption of the antibiotic was improved by some 2−3 fold over that of the parent compound. Recently the acyloxymethyl derivatization was extended to aminoacids such as α-methyl-DOPA (Saari *et al.*, 1978) or isoguvacine (Falch *et al.*, 1981).

Acylglycolic esters result from the reversal of the terminal ester group in acyloxymethyl esters (Fig. 6). Such compounds are known to be moderately activated esters and their possible use in peptide synthesis

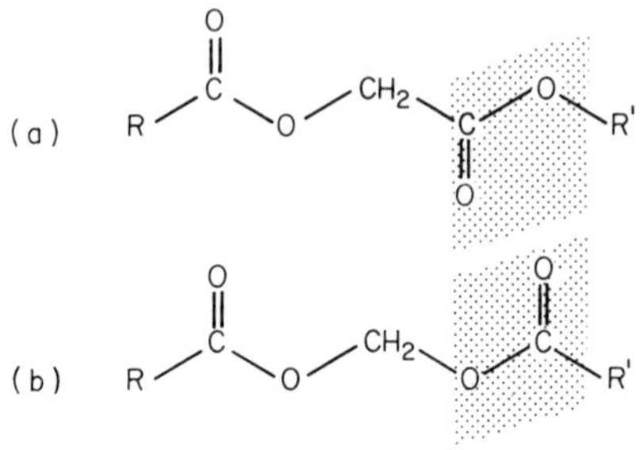

FIG. 6   Acylglycolic versus acyloxymethyl esters (Wermuth, 1980b)

was examined by Schwyzer and his group (1955a and b). Despite the fact that these compounds were claimed to be unsatisfactory candidates for the design of antibiotic prodrugs (Ferres, 1980), we decided to investigate their possible utility in the specific field of amino acid prodrugs. Acyloxymethyl esters of aspartic and glutamic acid showed some CNS stimulant activity which was not observed with the free acids (Wermuth, 1980b). The same approach, applied to the synthesis of the (-)-bornylglycolic prodrug of α-methyl-DOPA and some related compounds (Wermuth, 1978b), gave orally active derivatives which, on an equimolar basis, possess 2–3 times the potency of α-methyl-DOPA.

Hydrophilic carrier prodrugs
Water-solubility, starting from natural hydroxylic compounds is obtained by the use of the classical half-esters, hemisuccinates, hemiglutarates, hemiphthalates (Cocker *et al.*, 1965) or metasulphobenzoates (Allais *et al.*, 1962), which can give water soluble sodium, potassium or amine salts. However, given the facile hydrolysis of carboxylic esters of phenols, this method is not recommended for the solubilization of phenolic compounds. For these, as well as for alcohols, phosphoric esters constitute much better candidates. Phosphates have been used, particularly in the steroid (Flynn *et al.*, 1970; Melby *et al.*, 1961) and the vitamin field (Viscontini *et al.*, 1952; Ukita *et al.*, 1962). Clean phosphorylation methods are now available (Wermuth, 1981).

An alternative way to produce water-soluble prodrugs can be the synthesis of glycosides; for a review see Chavis and Imbach (1977). The β-glucoside of menthol represents an example of a non-irritating water soluble derivative of menthol (Higashiyama *et al.*, 1972).

British scientists from the Roche group recently described water-soluble prodrugs of 1,4-benzodiazepines (Hassal *et al.*, 1977). These compounds issued from a peptide bond formation between the open form of the benzodiazepine and a L-amino acid (preferentially L-lysine) (Fig. 7).

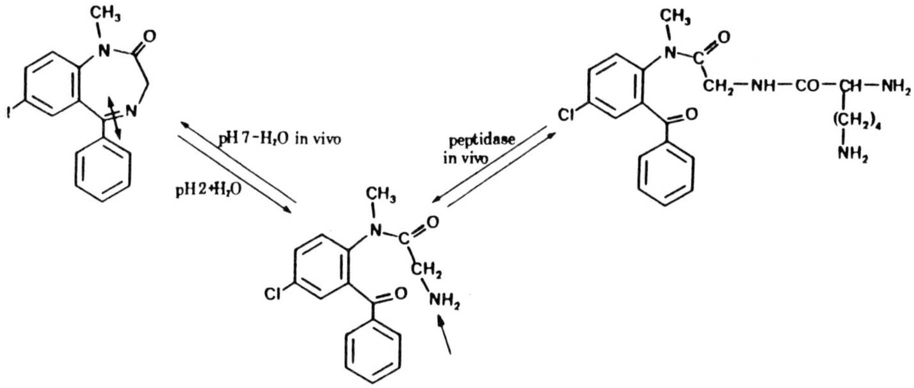

FIG. 7   Hydrosoluble prodrug of diazepam (Hassal *et al.*, 1977)

These prodrugs are freely soluble in water at the physiological pH of 7.4 and generate the active principle very rapidly *in vivo* after i.v. injection (2–3 minutes). The first step of the bioactivation is the hydrolysis of the peptide bond. The reaction is enzymatically catalysed and stereospecific, it does not occur when the terminal amino-acid is replaced by its non-natural D-antipode. The ring closure, however, is a purely chemical process, e.g. the half-life of the open form of diazepam is 73 seconds at pH 7. These water-soluble prodrugs of benzodiazepines represent a real progress in comparison with the propyleneglycol solutions which are potentially toxic (Martin and Finberg, 1970) or painful (Greenblatt *et al.*, 1974; Gamble *et al.*, 1973).

Site-selective delivery through carrier prodrugs

A selective renal vasodilatation is produced by administration of γ-glutamyl-DOPA. It is well known that L-DOPA is a precursor of the neurotransmitter substance dopamine, which plays an important role in the CNS and in the kidneys. The association of L-DOPA with a peripheral DOPA-decarboxylase inhibitor allows a preferential dopamine production in the brain and can be considered at present the best therapeutic possibility for Parkinson's disease.

On the renal side, a prodrug of L-DOPA, γ-glutamyl-L-3,4 dihydroxyphenylalanine (γ-glutamyl-DOPA), produces a specific vasodilatation of the renal tissue. Indeed, the γ-glutamyl derivatives of amino acids and peptides are accumulated in the kidneys where they undergo a selective metabolic process (for a review see Magnan *et al.*, 1982). The successive action of two enzymes present in high concentration in the kidney, γ-glutamyl transpeptidase and L-aromatic aminoacid decarboxylase, releases dopamine locally from γ-glutamyl-DOPA (Fig. 8).

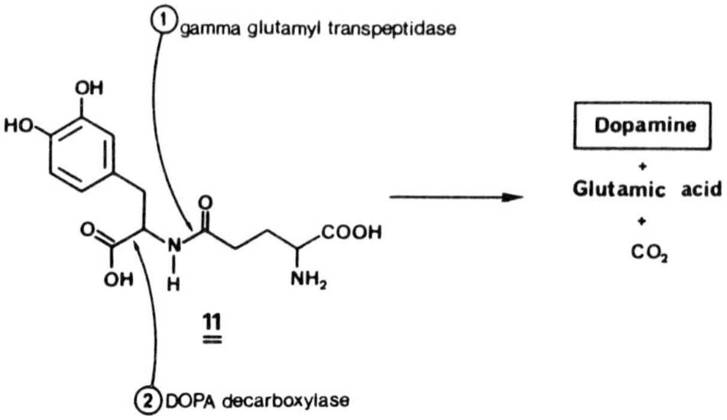

FIG. 8   Selective renal vasodilatation with γ-glutamyl-DOPA (Wilk *et al.*, 1978)

In mice, the renal levels of dopamine, after γ-glutamyl-DOPA administration, are five times higher than after an equimolar administration of L-DOPA. A perfusion of $10\mu M/g/30$ minutes of γ-glytamyl-DOPA in rats produces a 60% increase of the renal plasmatic flux (Wilk *et al.*, 1978). The same dose of L-DOPA induces no vasodilatation. Massive administration of γ-glutamyl-DOPA (20 times the preceeding dose) produces only a weak pressor effect, demonstrating that the systemic effects of the prodrug are low.

The same principle was utilized for the synthesis of γ-glutamyl derivatives of dopamine itself and diacyl-dopamines (Kyncl *et al.*, 1979; Jones *et al.*, 1977).

Prodrugs and chemical formulation problems

When the administration of a drug is associated with an uncomfortable or painful feeling it will find poor patient compliance and low medical prescriptions. The patient's refusal to take an orally given drug can be ascribed to its taste (bitterness, acidity, causticity) or its bad smell, but gastric irritations are also frequently invoked. Parenteral and rectal routes suppress some of these inconveniencies, but they often remain irritating and painful. Many prodrugs supposed to solve such problems have been described in the literature, although they will not be discussed here (Higuchi *et al.*, 1975; Roche, 1977; Wermuth, 1978a; Wermuth, 1980b).

A less frequent but interesting problem arises in the chemical modification of liquid active principles in solid prodrugs, suitable for tablet preparation. Figure 9, inspired by Stella (Higuchi *et al.*, 1975), indicates some chemical formulations of liquid active principles. The methodology often consists of the creation of symmetrical molecules presenting a higher tendency to crystallize.

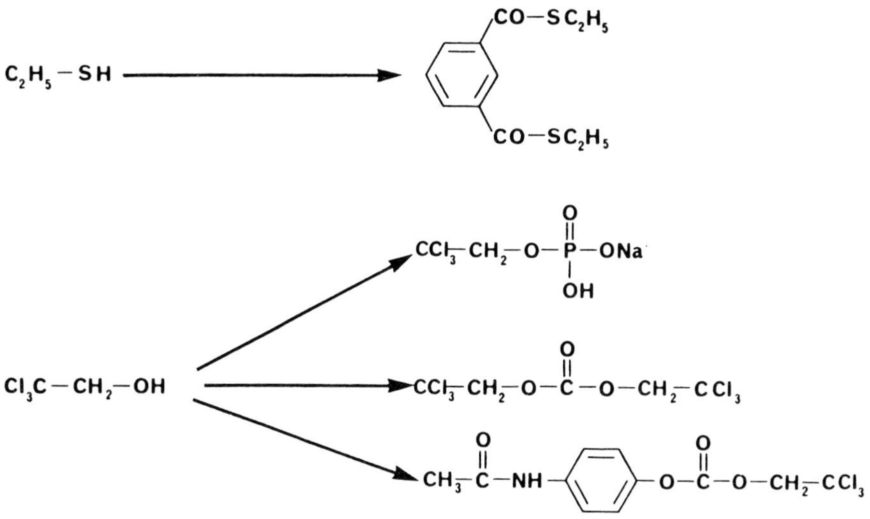

$C_2H_5-SH \longrightarrow$ [structure: benzene ring with two $CO-SC_2H_5$ groups]

Cl_3C-CH_2-OH [branches to three structures]

[top structure]
$$CCl_3-CH_2-O-\overset{\overset{\displaystyle O}{\|}}{P}-ONa$$
$\quad\quad\quad\quad\quad\quad OH$

[middle structure]
$$CCl_3-CH_2-O-\overset{\overset{\displaystyle O}{\|}}{C}-O-CH_2-CCl_3$$

[bottom structure]
$$CH_3-\overset{\overset{\displaystyle O}{\|}}{C}-NH-\text{[benzene ring]}-O-\overset{\overset{\displaystyle O}{\|}}{C}-O-CH_2-CCl_3$$

FIG. 9   Solid chemical formulations of liquid active principles (Higuchi and Stella, 1975)

Metabolic Precursors (Bioprecursors)

The Active Metabolite Concept

Since the pioneering experiments of the collaborators of Fourneau (Trefouël *et al.*, 1935) have demonstrated that Prontosil is inactive *in vitro* and is converted *in vivo* into sulphanilamide, the true active principle, the possibility of metabolic bioactivation was clearly recognized and largely developed, especially by Brodic (1964). Table 1 summarizes some early recognized active metabolites.

TABLE 1

Early recognized active metabolites

Drug	Active metabolite
Acetanilide	Paracetamol
Proguanil	Cycloguanil
Imipramine	Desmethylimipramine
Chloral hydrate	Trichloroethanol
Phenylbutazone	Oxyphenylbutazone
L-DOPA	Dopamine

Further metabolic studies made the distinction between phase I reactions which involve the transformation of specific groupings in a substrate molecule and the creation of new functional groups, and phase II reactions which are conjugations of the functions this created with convenient, mostly solubilizing, moieties (Testa and Jenner, 1976).

A survey of a great number of examples of active metabolites shows that they belong exclusively to the phase I products and result from one of the reactions mentioned in Table 2.

TABLE 2
Phase I Reactions (Testa *et al.*, 1976)

OXIDATIVE REACTIONS

Oxidation of alcohol, carbonyl, and acid functions, hydroxylation of aliphatic carbon atoms, hydroxylation of alicyclic carbon atoms, oxidation of aromatic carbon atoms, oxidation of carbon–carbon double bonds, oxidation of nitrogen-containing functional groups, oxidation of silicon, phosphorus, arsenic, and sulfur, oxidative *N*-dealkylation, oxidative *O*- and *S*-dealkylation, oxidative deamination, other oxidative reactions

REDUCTIVE REACTIONS

Reduction of carbonyl groups, reduction of alcoholic groups and carbon–carbon double bonds, reduction of nitrogen-containing functional groups, other reductive reactions

REACTIONS WITHOUT CHANGE IN THE STATE OF OXIDATION

Hydrolysis of esters and ethers, hydrolytic cleavage of C–N single bonds, hydrolytic cleavage of nonaromatic heterocycles, hydration and dehydration at multiple bonds, new atomic linkages resulting from dehydration reactions, hydrolytic dehalogenation: removal of hydrogen halide molecules, various reactions

As such reactions follow some general rules, they can often be forecasted. Taking into account the common metabolic pathways, one can imagine the design of a given molecule so that it will be converted *in vivo* into the desired compound by one or more of the phase I reactions. In other words the active metabolite concept can be used in a previsional way. The purpose of the following paragraphs is to illustrate some examples of design of this kind of prodrug for which we propose the name *bioprecursor*.

Designing Bioprecursors

The intentional use of bioprecursor design is relatively recent and in some cases there are some doubts on the prospective or the retrospective character of the design. Nevertheless, the following examples are presented to illustrate the variety of the approaches which can be utilized. The first examples relate to oxidative bioactivations, they are followed by examples of reductive bioactivations and finally by non-redox reactions. However, often the active species result from a cascade of metabolic reactions involving oxidative as well as reductive processes, complicated by hydrolytic reactions or hydration–dehydration sequences.

Pyrrolines as bioprecursors of GABA and GABA-analogues

A major obstacle in the design of potential therapeutic agents acting through the GABA system is the poor brain-penetration properties of active compounds. The approach taken by Callery *et al.* (1982) for the design of brain-penetrating compounds active on the GABA-system centres on the hypothesis that Δ^1-pyrroline and its analogues are bioprecursors of GABA and GABA-analogues (Fig. 10). This hypothesis is

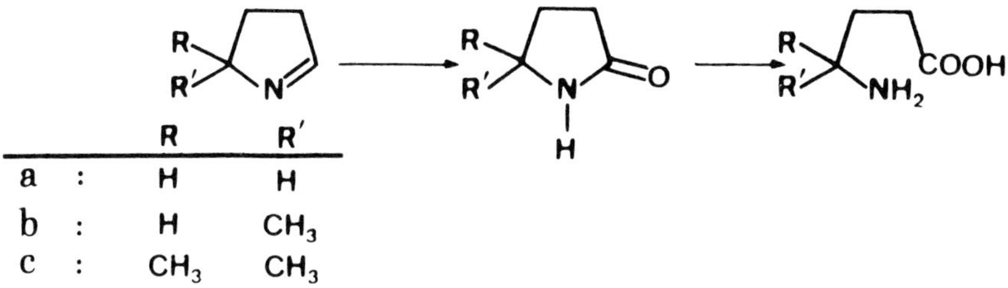

		R	R′
a	:	H	H
b	:	H	CH₃
c	:	CH₃	CH₃

FIG. 10   Pyrrolines as bioprecursors of GABA and GABA-analogues (Callery *et al.*, 1982)

inspired from the fact that putrescine was reported to be a precursor of GABA in mammalian systems (Tabor and Tabor, 1964) and that the proposed pathway (Fig. 11) involves the conversion of Δ^1-pyrroline to GABA.

The capacity of brain tissue to carry out this conversion was demonstrated by *in vivo* brain studies. After an intraperitoneal injection of

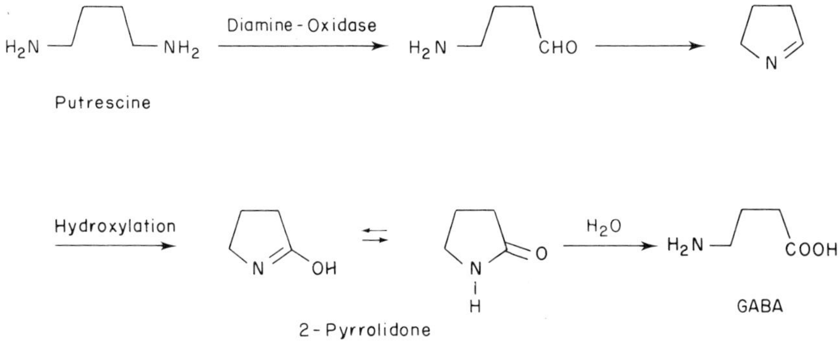

FIG. 11   The metabolism of putrescine (Tabor and Tabor, 1964)

200 mg/kg of 5-methyl-Δ^1-pyrroline to mice, the brain concentrations for 4-methyl-GABA were 170 and 270 μM, 0.5 and 5 hours respectively after administration. These levels exceed by far the IC_{50} value of 3.5 μM reported for inhibition of GABA-binding *in vitro* by 4-methyl-GABA (Iversen *et al.*, 1978). On the other hand, 4-methyl-GABA did not penetrate the central nervous system in measurable quantities following intraperitoneal administration to mice in high doses (400 mg/kg).

Site-specific delivery of the acetylcholine-esterase reactivator 2-PAM to the brain

N-methylpyridinium-2-carbaldoxime (2-PAM) (a) constitutes the most potent reactivator of acetylcholinesterase poisoned through organophosphorus acylation. However, due to its quaternary nitrogen, 2-PAM penetrates very poorly the biological membranes and does not appreciably cross the blood–brain barrier. For this compound Bodor *et al.* (1976) designed an ingenious dihydropyridine-pyridinium salt type of redox delivery system. The active drug is administered as its 5,6-dihydropyridine derivative (Pro-2-PAM) (b), which exists as a stable immonium salt (c). The lipoidal (b) ($pK_a = 6.32$) easily penetrates the blood–brain barrier where it is oxidized to the active (a) (Fig. 12).

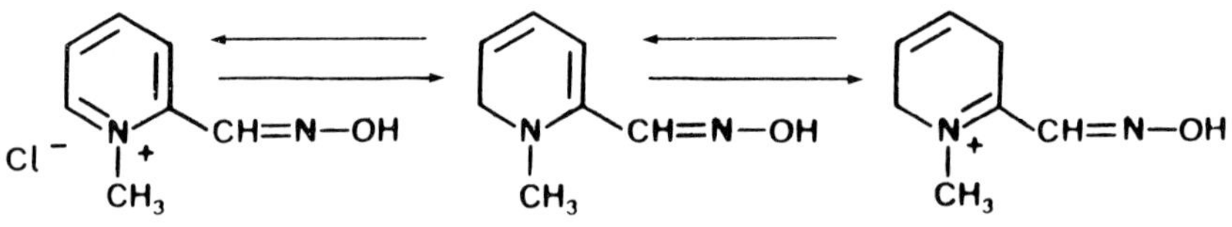

FIG. 12   Dihydro derivatives of 2-PAM (Bodor *et al.*, 1976)

A dramatic increase in the brain delivery of 2-PAM by the use of Pro-2-PAM was thus achieved, resulting in a re-activation of phosphorylated brain acetylcholinesterase *in vivo* (Shek *et al.*, 1976 and Shek and Higuchi, 1976).

Conversion of N-alkylaminobenzophenones to benzodiazepines 'in vivo'

N-dealkylation of tertiary amines is a very frequently encountered metabolic process (Testa and Jenner, 1976) and may be successfully used in bioprecursor design. A practical example is found in the case of N-alkylaminobenzophenones, which are open ring analogues of the corresponding benzodiazepines (Gall *et al.*, 1976). These compounds possess potent sedative and muscle relaxing activities and, in addition, antagonize pentylenetetrazole-induced clonic convulsions. It was demonstrated (Lahti and Gall, 1976) that, *in vivo*, they undergo *N*-dealkylation and ring closure to form the corresponding benzodiazepine (Fig. 13). The *in vivo* conversion was found to occur in mice, rats and monkeys. These findings suggest that their observed pharmacological

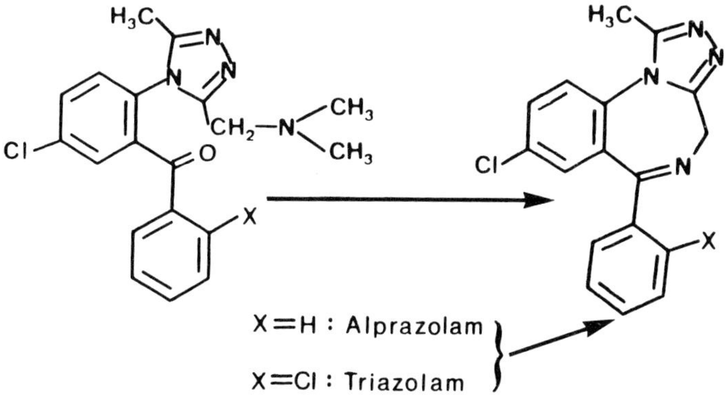

X=H : Alprazolam

X=Cl : Triazolam

FIG. 13 Conversion of *N*-alkylaminobenzophenones to benzodiazepines *in vivo* (Lahti and Gall, 1976)

activity may be due to the formation of the corresponding benzodiazepine. The conversion was actually confirmed by a comparison of retention times on a gas chromatograph as well as through the use of GC-mass spectrometer.

Reductive bioactivation of sulindac
Sulindac, *cis*-5-fluoro-2-methyl-1-(p-(methylsulphinyl) benzylidene) indene-3 acetic acid (Shen *et al.*, 1972), is a nonsteroidal anti-inflammatory agent having a broad spectrum of activity in animal models and in man. The two quantitatively significant biotransformations undergone by sulindac in laboratory species (Hucker *et al.*, 1973) and in man (Duggan *et al.*, 1977a) involve only changes in the oxidation state of the sulphinyl substituent, viz., oxidation of the parent (sulindac) to sulphone and reduction to sulphide (Fig. 14), the latter being the active species (Duggan *et al.*, 1977b). In two *in vitro* models of inflammation, prostaglandin synthetase inhibition and inhibition of platelet aggregation, the sulphide has activities comparable to those of indomethacin, whereas sulindac itself is devoid of activity.

Nevertheless, sulindac is the preferred compound for clinical applications: an oral dosage of this inactive bioprecursor will circumvent initial exposure of gastric and intestinal mucosa to the active drug,

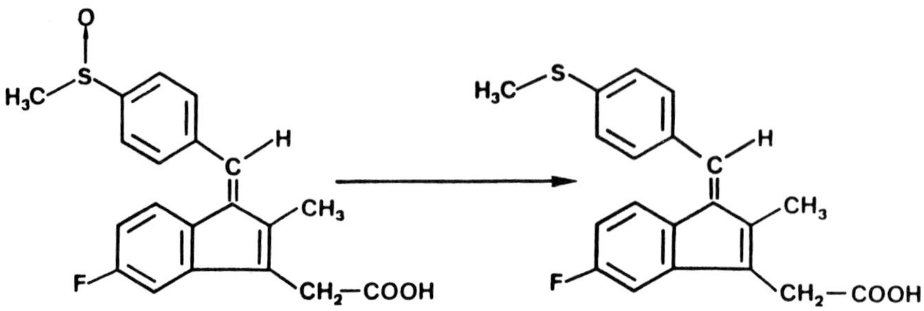

FIG. 14   Reductive bioactivation of sulindac (Duggan *et al.*, 1977b)

and might thus provide a therapeutic advantage relative to dosing with the sulphide.

The bioreductive alkylation concept

This concept of bioreductive alkylation was put forth by Lin, Cosby, Shansky and Sartorelli (1972). The challenge is to design a biologically inactive form of the compounds which become potent alkylating agents after *in vivo* reduction. One of the models proposed by Sartorelli, Lin and co-workers (Lin *et al.*, 1972, 1973, 1975; Lin and Sartorelli, 1973) is that of simple quinone methides (Fig. 15). Certain simple quinones

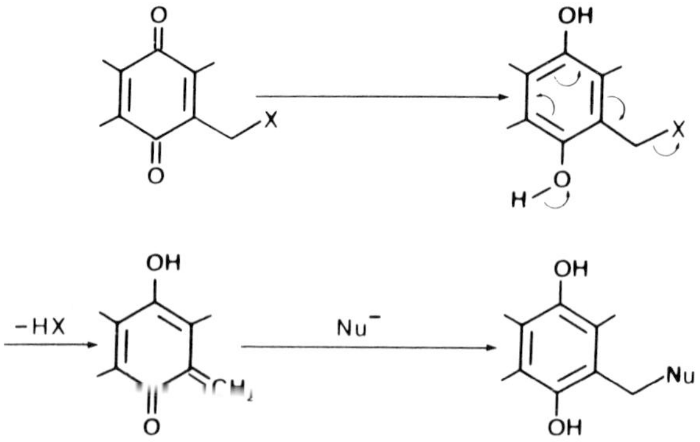

FIG. 15   The bioreductive alkylation concept (Moore, 1977)

substituted by one (or more) -CH$_2$-X groups present marked antineoplastic activity. These compounds may function as alkylating agents after reduction to the corresponding hydroquinones which in turn yield quinone methides, the key alkylating agents *in vivo*.

In a review article, Moore (1977) discussed the concept of bioreductive alkylation as the mechanism of action of many naturally occurring and synthetic antitumour agents and antibiotics. Four models are presented (activated enamines, vinylogous quinone methides, simple quinone methides and α-methylene lactones or lactams). They may account for the activity of a large number of well-known agents: mitomycin, doxorubicin, daunorubicin, camptothecin, etc.

Arylacetic acids from aroylpropionic precursors
A careful examination of the metabolic pathways involved in the biotransformation of nicotine and haloperidol clearly indicates the existence of a progressive degradation of the aroylpropionic side-chain into arylacetic acids (Testa and Jenner, 1976) (Fig. 16).

This information was utilized to design bucloxic acid (Krausz *et al.*, 1974; Gros *et al.*, 1974), fenbufene (Kohler *et al.*, 1980; Chiccarelli *et al.*, 1980) and furobufene (Martel *et al.*, 1974) which are all three bioprecursor-forms of anti-inflammatory arylacetic acids (Fig. 17). For all these compounds the bioactivation takes place through a multistep process implying reductive, oxidative and hydration – dehydration sequences.

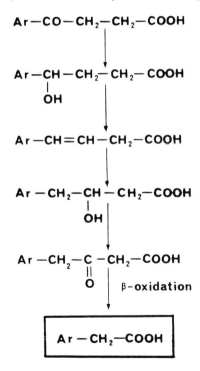

FIG. 16   Progressive metabolic degradation of β-aroylpropionic acid into arylacetic acid (Testa and Jenner, 1976)

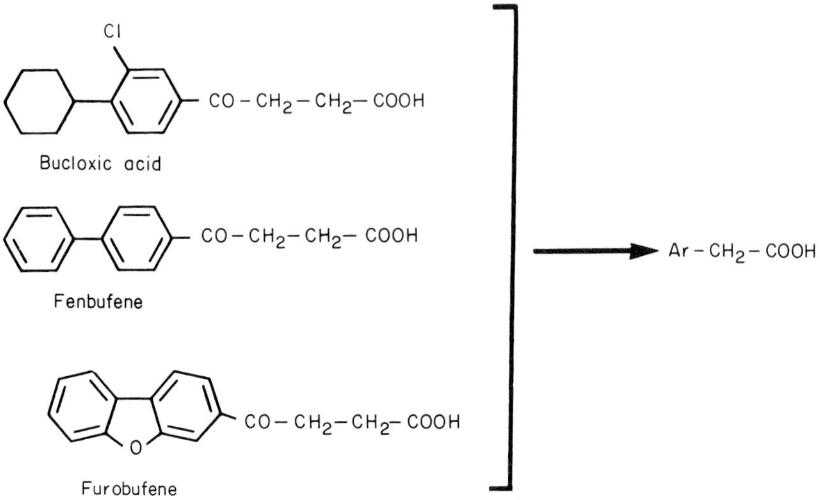
Cl
CO – CH2 – CH2 – COOH
Bucloxic acid
CO – CH2 – CH2 – COOH
Fenbufene
CO – CH2 – CH2 – COOH
O
Furobufene
Ar – CH2 – COOH

FIG. 17 Anti-inflammatory agents presenting the aroylpropionic structure (Krausz *et al.*, 1974; Kohler *et al.*, 1980; Martel *et al.*, 1974)

L-2-oxothiazolidine-4-carboxylate: a cysteine delivery system

The enzyme 5-oxo-L-prolinase that catalyses the conversion of 5-oxo-L-proline to L-glutamate coupled to the consumption of ATP (Fig. 18) was shown by Williamson and Meister (1981) to act also on a synthetic substrate, L-2-oxothiazolidine-4-carboxylate, which is an analogue of 5-oxoproline in which the 4-methylene group is replaced by sulphur.

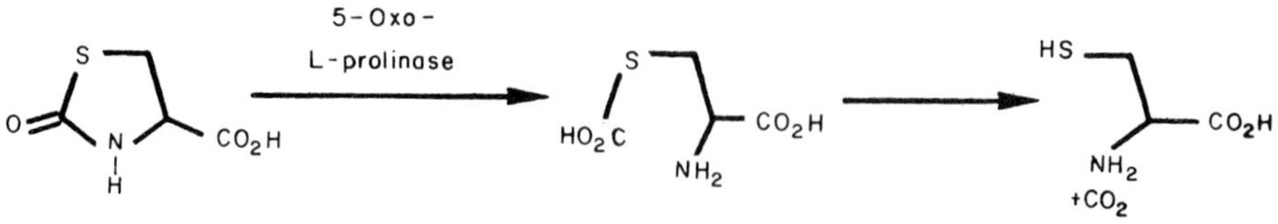
S
O
N
H
CO2H
5-Oxo-
L-prolinase
S
HO2C
NH2
CO2H
HS
NH2
+CO2
CO2H

FIG. 18 L-2-oxothiazolidine-4-carboxylate: an intracellular cysteine delivery system (Williamson and Meister, 1981)

The enzyme, which exhibits a similar affinity for the analogue and the natural substrate, is inhibited by the analogue *in vitro* and *in vivo*. L-3-oxothiazolidine-4-carboxylate thus serves as a potent inhibitor of the γ-glutamyl cycle at the step of 5-oxoprolinase. Administration of L-2-oxothiazolidine-4-carboxylate to mice deprived of hepatic glutathione led to restoration of normal hepatic glutathione levels. Since L-2-oxothiazoline-4 carboxylate is an excellent substrate of the enzyme, it may serve as an intracellular delivery system for cysteine and thus a potential as a therapeutic agent for conditions in which there is depletion of hepatic glutathione.

Intracellular delivery of phenylglyoxylic acids
In the context of ischemic heart disease, particularly following myocardial infarction, the stimulation of the multi-enzyme complex pyruvate dehydrogenase (PDH) offers a means of "switching over" myocardial metabolism from fatty acid utilization to glucose, which is more economical in terms of oxygen consumption (Neely and Morgan, 1974). Amongst the agents able to promote carbohydrate oxidation by increasing PDH levels in the heart, α-keto-acids, and especially phenylglyoxylic acids, proved to be valuable candidates (Barnish *et al.*, 1981). Attempts to increase the *in vivo* activity of p-hydroxy-phenyl-glyoxylic acid and to prolong the duration of its action by delivering them into cells as prodrug, suggested the use of L-(+)-2-(4-hydroxyphenyl) glycine or oxfenicine (Fig. 19) (Barnish *et al.*, 1981). Effectively, amino acids are known to be transported across lipid membranes by an active transport process. In addition, it is known that L-(+)-α-amino acids are converted to α-keto acids by transaminase enzymes.

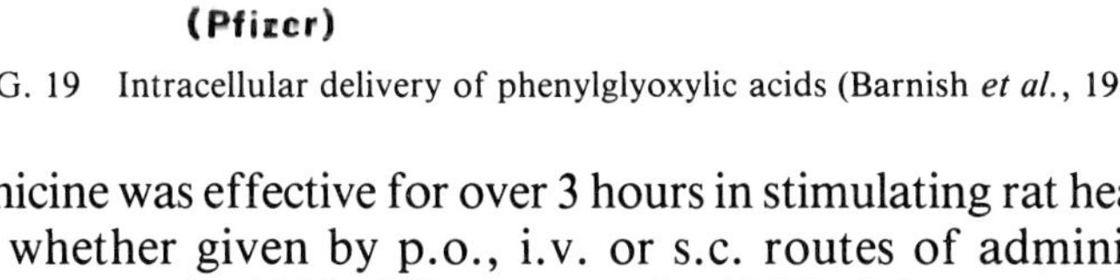

Oxfenicin

(Pfizer)

FIG. 19   Intracellular delivery of phenylglyoxylic acids (Barnish *et al.*, 1981)

Oxfenicine was effective for over 3 hours in stimulating rat heart PDH activity whether given by p.o., i.v. or s.c. routes of administration (Blackburn *et al.*, 1979; Higgins *et al.*, 1980). Moreover, pharmacokinetic studies in rats, dogs and man have shown that p-hydroxy-phenylglyoxylic acid appears in the blood soon after administration of oxfenicine. Oxfenicine is presently undergoing clinical trials for ischemic heart disease.

Discussion

Bioprecursors Versus Carrier-Prodrugs

A comparative balance-sheet established for the two prodrug approaches led us to the following conclusions (Table 3):

The *bioavailability* of carrier-prodrugs is modulated by using a transient transport moiety; such a linkage is not implied for bioprecursors which result from a molecular modification of the active principle itself.

The *lipophilicity* is generally the subject of a profound alteration of the parent molecule in the case of carrier-prodrugs, whereas it remains practically unchanged for bioprecursors.

The *bioactivation* process is exclusively hydrolytic for carrier-prodrugs; it involves mostly redox systems for bioprecursors.

The *catalysis* leading to the active principle is hydrolytic (either through general catalysis or through extra-hepatic enzymes) for carrier-prodrugs. For bioprecursors, it seems rather restricted to phase I metabolizing enzymes.

TABLE 3

Bioprecursors versus carrier-prodrugs

| | Prodrugs | |
	Carrier prodrugs	Bioprecursors
Constitution	Active principle + carrier group	No carrier group
Lipophilicity	Strongly modified	Slightly modified
Bioactivation	Hydrolytic	Oxidative or reductive
Catalysis	Chemical or enzymic	Only enzymic

Existence of Mixed-Type of Prodrugs

In some cases the design of mixed-type prodrugs can be advantageous as illustrated in the following two examples.

Disulphide thiamine prodrugs

Compounds like (a) and (b) result from lipophilic disulphide derivation of the open ring thiolate anion corresponding to thiamine (Fig. 20) (Matsukawa *et al.*, 1962). Such compounds can also be considered as carrier-prodrugs, in so far as the thiolate is linked to a n-propylthio (a) or a tetrahydrofuranyl-methylenethio (b) transport moiety, or as bioprecursors, in so far as a bioreductive cleavage into the thiolate anion is needed to generate the active thiamine; the thiolate anion then

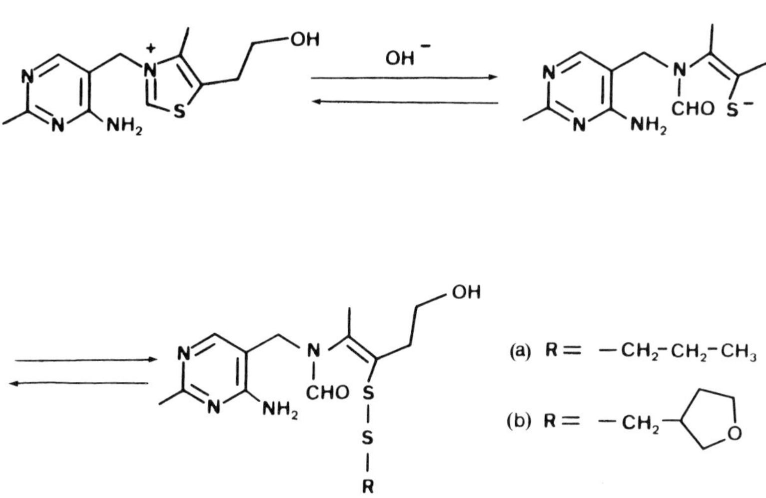

FIG. 20   Disulphide thiamine prodrugs as example of mixed-type prodrugs (Matsukawa *et al.*, 1962)

functions as a less polar (no quaternary ammonium function) precursor form of thiamine.

Trigonelline esters and amides
Generalizing the dihydropyridine ⇌ pyridinium salt redox delivery system, successfully applied to 2-PAM, Bodor and his co-workers (1981) proposed an astute sustained release methodology for brain delivery, based on the mixed-type prodrugs.
The biologically active compound is linked to a lipoidal dihydropyridine carrier which easily penetrates the blood–brain barrier (Fig. 21). Enzymatic oxidation *in vivo* by the NAD ⇌ NADH system of the carrier part to the ionic pyridinium salt prevents its elimination from the brain, while elimination from the general circulation is accelerated. Subsequent cleavage of the quaternary carrier-drug species results in sustained delivery of the drug in the brain and a facile elimination of the non-toxic carrier part (trigonelline or its *N*-benzyl analogue).

Difficulties and Limitations

The introduction of prodrugs in human therapy indeed gave successful results in overcoming undesirable properties such as poor absorption, too fast biodegradation, or various formulation problems. It can be expected that an increasing number of medicinal chemists will be

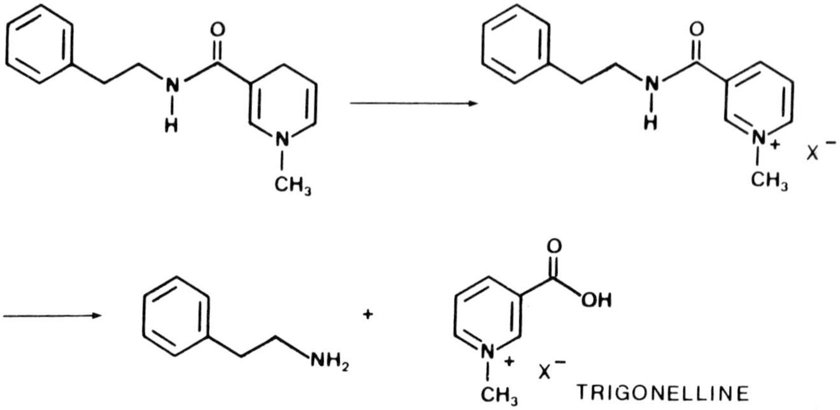

FIG. 21   Trigonelline esters and amides as example of mixed-type prodrugs (Bodor *et al.*, 1981)

tempted by this approach. However, they must keep in mind that pro-drug design can also give rise to a large number of new difficulties, especially in the assessment of their pharmacological, pharmacokinetic, toxicological and clinical properties.

At the *pharmacological level*, for example, due to the necessity of bioactivation to create the active species, these compounds cannot be submitted to preliminary *in vitro* screening tests, namely, binding studies, neurotransmitter re-uptake, measurements of enzymatic in-hibition and activity on isolated organs.

The measurements of *pharmacokinetic parameters* can give rise to numerous misinterpretations. Thus pivampicillin has a half-life of 103 minutes in a buffered aqueous solution at 37°C, but it falls to less than one minute after addition of only 1% of mouse or rat serum. In the presence of human serum (10%) however, it is 50 minutes, whereas in whole human blood it is only 5 minutes. These results exemplify how careful one must be in investigating such experiments to avoid incorrect conclusions. In addition, when a prodrug and the parent molecule are compared, one must take into account the differences in their respective time courses of action. The maximum activity can appear later for the prodrug than for the parent compound, and often the comparison of the area under the curve could constitute a better criterion.

At the *toxicological level*, even when they derive from well-known active principles, prodrugs have to be regarded as new entities. Un-desirable side-effects can appear which are directly related to the prodrug (allergy to bucloxic acid) or derived from the bioactivation process (formation of unwanted or unexpected metabolites) or which can be attributed to the temporary transport moiety (digestive intolerance to pivampicillin, antivitamin-PP activity of nicaphenine due to the hydro-xyethylnicotinamide carrier group etc.).

In a recent review of potential hazards of the prodrug approach, Gorrod (1980) cites four toxicity mechanisms:

1) Formation of a toxic metabolite of the total prodrug, which is not produced by the parent drug.
2) Consumption of a vital constituent (for example glutathione) during the prodrug activation process.
3) Generation of a toxic derivative from a transport moiety supposed to be "inert".
4) Release of a pharmacokinetic modifier (causing enzymatic induction, displacing protein-bound molecules, altering drug excretion, etc.).

At the *clinical stage* eventually, the predictive value of animal experiments is also questionable. Thus, for two prodrugs derived from α-methyl-DOPA, the active doses in the rat were identical; nonetheless, they turned out to be very different during the clinical investigations. One compound was just as active as α-methyl-DOPA, whereas the other one was 3 − 4 times more active (Saari *et al.*, 1978; Vickers *et al.*, 1978).

An application file for a new prodrug should take into account all these aspects and can in no way be regarded just as a complement to the main file.

Conclusion

In the future it would be preferable to distinguish clearly the carrier-prodrug and the bioprecursor approaches. The first one, consisting in the attachment of a temporary carrier group to an active principle, largely proved its utility in the design of orally active antibiotics and more generally every time high bioavailability in plasma or peripheral organs is required. The CNS delivery of drugs by the use of carrier-prodrugs, is less convincing in that usually high dosages are needed to ascertain clinical efficiency (1 − 2 g progabide per day, for example).

The design of bioprecursors, which represents a creative application of the active metabolite concept in the previsional way seems *a priori* more adequate for CNS delivery, but it still has to prove the reality of its clinical usefulness.

Mixed-type approaches gave good results for thiamine and appear to be an interesting alternative when each individual approach fails.

References

Akesson, B., Gronowitz, S., Herslof, B. and Ohlson, R. (1978). *Lipids* 13, 338–343.

Albert, A. (1958). *Nature (London)* 182, 421–423.

Albert, A. (1964). "Selective Toxicity". Chapman and Hall, London.

Allais, A. and Girault, P. (1962). U.S. Patent 3,032,568 May 1, 1961 (Roussel-Uclaf, S.A.).

Anden, N.E., Corrodi, H., Dahlström, A., Fuxe, K. and Hokfelt, T. (1966). *Life Sci.* 5, 561–568.

Barnish, I.T., Cross, E.P., Danilewicz, J.C., Dickinson, R.P. and Stopher, D.A. (1981). *J. Med. Chem.* 24, 399–404.

Binderup, E., Godtfredsen, W.O. and Roholt, K. (1971). *J. Antibiot.* 24, 767–773.

Blackburn, K.J., Burges, R.A., Gardiner, D.G., Higgins, A.J., Morville, M. and Page, M.G. (1979). *Br. J. Pharmacol.* 66, 443P–444P.

Bodin, N.O., Ekström, B., Forsgren, U., Jular, L.P., Magni, L., Ramsey, C.H. and Sjöberg, B. (1975). *Antimicrob. Agents Chemother.* 8 (5), 518–525.

Bodor, N., Shek, E. and Higuchi, T. (1976). *J. Med. Chem.* 19, 102–107.

Bodor, N., Farag, H.H. and Brewster III, M.E. (1981). *Science* 214, 1370–1372.

Brodie, B.B. (1964). *In* "Actualités Pharmacologiques, 17ème série" (R. Hazard and J. Cheymol, eds), pp. 1–40. Masson et Cie, Paris.

Callery, P.S., Geelhaar, L.A., Nayar, B.M.S., Stogniew, M. and Rao, K.G. (1982). *J. Neurochem.* 38, 1063–1067.

Chavis, C. and Imbach, J.L. (1977). *In* "Actualités de Chimie Thérapeutique: 5ème série", pp. 3–28. Société de Chimie Thérapeutique, Châtenay-Malabry, France.

Chiccarelli, F.S., Eisner, H.J. and Van Lear, G.E. (1980). *Arzneim. Forsch.* 30, 707–715.

Clayton, J.P., Cole, M., Elson, S.W., Ferres, H., Hanson, J.C., Mizen, L.W. and Sutherland, R. (1976). *J. Med. Chem.* 19, 1385–1391.

Cocker, J.D., Elks, J., May, P.J., Nice, F.A., Phillipps, G.H. and Wall, W.F. (1965). *J. Med. Chem.* 8, 417–425.

Daehne, W. von, Frederiksen, E., Gundersen, E., Lund, F., March, P., Petersen, H.J., Roholt, K., Tybring, L. and Godtfredsen, W.O. (1970). *J. Med. Chem.* 13, 607–612.

Duggan, D.E., Hare, L.E., Ditzler, C.A., Lei, B.W. and Kwan, K.C. (1977a). *Clin. Pharmacol. Ther.* 21, 326–335.

Duggan, D.E., Hooke, K.F., Risley, E.A., Shen, T.Y. and Van Arman, C.G. (1977b). *J. Pharmacol. Exp. Ther.* 201, 8–13.

Falch, E., Krogsgaard-Larsen, P. and Christensen, A.V. (1981). *J. Med. Chem.* 24, 285–289.

Falconi, G., Galletti, F., Celasco, G. and Gardi, R. (1972). *Steroids* 20, 627–632.

Ferron, H. (1980). *Chem. Ind. (London)*, 436–440.

Flynn, G.L. and Lamb, D.J. (1970). *J. Pharm. Sci.* 59, 1433–1438.

Frey, H.H., Popp, C. and Löscher, W. (1979). *Neuropharmacology* 18, 581–590.

Gall, M., Hester, J.B. Jr, Rudzik, A.D. and Lahti, R.A. (1976). *J. Med. Chem.* 19, 1057–1064.

Gamble, J.A.S., Mac Kay, J.S. and Dundee, J.W. (1973). *Br. J. Anaesth.* 45, 1085.

Gorrod, J.W. (1980). *Chem. Ind. (London)*, 457–461.

Greenblatt, D.J., Shader, R.I. and Koch-Weser, J. (1974). *N. Engl. J. Med.* 291, 1116–1118.

Gros, P.M., Davi, H.J., Chasseaud, L.F. and Hawkins, D.R. (1974). *Arzneim. Forsch.* 24, 1385–1390.

Harper, N.J. (1959). *J. Med. Pharm. Chem.* 1, 467–500.

Hassal, C.H., Holmes, S.W., Johnson, W.H., Kröhn, A., Smithen, C.E. and Thomas, W.A. (1977). *Experientia* 33, 1492–1493.

Higashiyama, T. and Sakata, I. (1972). Ger. Offen. 2 242 237, 28 August 1972 (Kasaoka, Okayama, Japan).

Higgins, A.J., Burges, R.A., Gardiner, D.G., Morville, M., Page, M.G. and Blackburn, K.J. (1980). *Life Sci.* 27, 963–970.

Higuchi, T. and Stella, V. (1975). "Pro-drugs as a Novel Drug Delivery Systems". American Chemical Society, Washington.

Horn, A.S. (1980). *Chem. Ind. (London)*, 441–444.

Hucker, H.B., Stauffer, S.C., White, S.D., Rhodes, R.E., Arison, B.H., Umbenhauer, E.F., Bower, R.J. and McMahon, F.G. (1973). *Drug Metab. Dispos.* 1, 721–736.

Iversen, L.L., Bird, E., Spokes, E., Nicholson, S.H. and Suckling, C.J. (1978). *In* "Agonist Specificity of GABA Binding Sites in Human Brain and GABA in Huntington's Disease and Schizophrenia". GABA Neurotransmitters (P. Kroogsgaard-Larsen, J. Scheel-Krüger and H. Kofod, eds), pp. 179–190. Academic Press, New York.

Jansen, A.B.A. and Russel, T.J. (1965). *J. Chem. Soc.*, 2127–2132.

Jones, G. (1980). *Chem. Ind. (London)*, 452–456.

Jones, P.H., Kyncl, J., Ours, C.W. and Somani, P. (1977). United States Patent 4.017.636 Apr. 12, 1977 (Abott Laboratories).

Kohler, C., Tolman, E., Wooding, W. and Ellenbogen, L. (1980). *Arzneim. Forsch.* 30, 702–707.

Krausz, F., Demarne, H., Vaillant, J., Brunaud, M. and Navarro, J. (1974). *Arzneim. Forsch.* 24 (9a), 1360–1364.

Kyncl, J.J., Minard, F.N. and Jones, P.H. (1979). *In* "Symposium on Peripheral Dopaminergic Receptors". Strasbourg, July 1978. (J.L. Imbs and J. Schwartz, eds), pp. 353–364. Pergamon Press, Oxford.

Lahti, R.A. and Gall, M. (1976). *J. Med. Chem.* 19, 1064–1067.

Lin, A.J., Cosby, L.A., Shansky, C.W. and Sartorelli, A.C. (1972). *J. Med. Chem.* 15, 1247–1252.

Lin, A.J., Pardini, R.S., Cosby, L.A., Lillis, B.J., Shansky, C.W. and Sartorelli, A.C. (1973). *J. Med. Chem.* 16, 1268–1276.

Lin, A.J. and Sartorelli, A.C. (1973). *J. Org. Chem* 38, 813–815.

Lin, A.J., Lillis, B.J. and Sartorelli, A.C. (1975). *J. Med. Chem.* 18, 917–921.

McClure, D. (1975). *In* "Pro-drugs as a Novel Drug Delivery Systems" (T. Higuchi and V. Stella, eds), pp. 224–234. American Chemical Society, Washington.

Magnan, S.D.J., Shirota, F.N. and Nagasawa, H.T. (1982). *J. Med. Chem.* 25, 1018–1021.

Martel, R.R., Rochefort, J.G., Klicius, J. and Dobson, T.A. (1974). *Can. J. Physiol. Pharmacol.* 52, 669–673.

Martin, G. and Finsberg, L. (1970). *J. Pediatr.* 77, 877–878.

Matsukawa, T., Yurugi, S. and Oka, Y. (1962). *Ann. N.Y. Acad. Sci.* 98, 430–444.

Melby, J.C. and St. Cyr, M. (1961). *Metabolism* 10, 75–82.

Moore, H.W. (1977). *Science* 197, 527–532.

Neely, J.R. and Morgan, H.E. (1974). *Annu. Rev. Physiol.* 36, 413–459.

Ostrovskaya, R.U., Parin, V.V. and Tsybina, N.M. (1972). *Byull. Eksp. Biol. Med.* 1, 51–55.

Roche, B. (1977). "Design of Biopharmaceutical Properties through Prodrugs and Analogs". American Pharmaceutical Association, Washington.

Saari, W.S., Freedman, M.B., Hartman, R.D., King, S.W., Raab, A.W., Randall, W.C., Engelhart, E.L., Hirschmann, R., Rosegay, A., Ludden, C.T. and Scriabine, A. (1978). *J. Med. Chem.* 21, 746–753.

72   C.G. Wermuth

Schwyzer, R., Iselin, B. and Feurer, M. (1955a). *Helv. Chim. Acta* **38**, 69–79.
Schwyzer, R., Feurer, M., Iselin, B. and Kägi, H. (1955b). *Helv. Chim. Acta* **38**, 80–83.
Shek, E. and Higuchi, T. (1976a). *J. Med. Chem.* **19**, 113–117.
Shek, E., Higuchi, T. and Bodor, N. (1976b). *J. Med. Chem.* **19**, 108–112.
Shen, T.Y., Witzel, B.E., Jones, H., Linn, B.O., McPherson, J., Greenwald, R., Fordice, M. and Jacob, A. (1972). *Fed. Proc. Fed. Am. Soc. Exp. Biol.* **31**, 577.
Sinkula, A.A. (1977). *In* "Medicinal Chemistry" (J. Mathieu, ed.), Vol. V, 125–133. Elsevier, Amsterdam.
Tabor, H. and Tabor, C.W. (1964). *Pharmacol. Rev.* **16**, 245–300.
Testa, B. and Jenner, P. (1976). "Drug Metabolism, Chemical and Biochemical Aspects". Marcel Dekker, New York.
Trefouël, J., Trefouël, T., Nitti, F. and Bovet, D. (1935). *C.R. Séances Soc. Biol.* **120**, 756–758.
Tsibina, N.M., Ostrovskaya, R.U., Protopova, T.V., Parin, V.V., Selezneva, N.I. and Skolainov, A.P. (1974). *Khim. Farm. Zh.* **17**, 10–13.
Ukita, C. and Nagazawa, K. (1962). Japan Patent 23 014, Nov. 28, 1961 (Takeda Chemical Industries, Ltd.); *Chem. Abstr.* **57**, 16729 d.
Vickers, S., Duncan, C.A., White, S.D., Breault, G.O., Boyds, R.B., de Shepper, P.J. and Tempero, K.F. (1978). *Drug Metabolism and Disposition* **6**, 640–646.
Viscontini, H., Ebnöther, C. and Karrer, P. (1952). *Helv. Chim. Acta* **35**, 457–459.
Wermuth, C.G. (1978a). *Pour la Science* (Scientific American, French Edition) **2**, 47–61.
Wermuth, C.G. (1978b). *Ger. Offen 2,743,166* Mar. 30, 1978 (Synthelabo S.A.); *Chem. Abstr.* **89**, 110,405f.
Wermuth, C.G. (1980a). *Bull. Soc. Pharm. Bordeaux* **119**, 107–129.
Wermuth, C.G. (1980b). *Chem. Ind. (London)*, 433–435.
Wermuth, C.G. (1981). *In* "Natural Products as Medicinal Agents" (J.L. Beal and E. Reinhard, eds), pp. 185–216, Hippokrates Verlag, Stuttgart.
Wermuth, C.G. (1983). *In* "Drug Metabolism and Drug Design: Quo Vardis?" (M. Briot, W. Cautreels and R. Roncucci, eds). Sanofi-Clin-Midy, Montpellier.
Wilk, S., Mizoguchi, H. and Orlowski, M. (1978). *J. Pharmacol. Exp. Ther.* **206**, 227–232.
Williamson, J.M. and Meister, A. (1981). *Proc. Natl. Acad. Sci. U.S.A.* **78**, 936–939.

5 Statistics and Drug Design

S. CLEMENTI

Dipartimento di Chimica, Universita' di Perugia,
Via Elce di Sotto, 10-06100 Perugia, Italy

Introduction

Chemometrics is the new discipline which studies the application of mathematical and statistical methods in various branches of chemistry (Kowalski and Bender, 1972). Its recent development was made possible by the wider and easier access to computing facilities over the last decade. In particular, multivariate statistics has proved to be very valuable for handling complex problems in natural sciences (Wold, 1983).

Why should multivariate statistics be relevant to drug design? Let us state that the final goal in this area is the synthesis of a chemical compound with certain optimal features, in the absence of undesired effects, in its biological activity. In this case the multivariate statistical approach is the best possible tool to be used, since it is the best way of utilizing all the information required at the same time. The various multivariate methods are indeed aimed at describing the structure of the available data set and therefore at predicting the behaviour of new samples. Accordingly, they are clearly suitable for coping with drug design problems (Dunn *et al.*, 1978; Dunn and Wold; 1978a; Dunn and Wold, 1978b; Dunn and Wold, 1980b; Dunn and Wold, 1981).

Chemometrics is usually defined as consisting of two main objectives: (a) the optimization of experimental procedures, and (b) the extraction

DRUG DESIGN: FACT OR FANTASY
ISBN 0.12.388180.3

of chemical information contained in a data set (Massart *et al.*, 1978). Both these studies are relevant to drug design. The former approach, requiring an appropriate experimental design to detect the importance of individual variables, allows the construction of isoresponse plots (Box *et al.*, 1978). Such methods are becoming increasingly useful in organic synthesis. However, the second approach, which in principle also permits the interpretation of the causes of a biological response, is more common and widely used in literature work especially in the area of quantitative structure–activity relationships (QSAR). The scope of this paper is to review critically the most popular such methods and to summarize a few preliminary results from our laboratory.

Multivariate Statistics

A data set suitable for a multivariate analysis consists of a table (matrix) where a number (M) of manifest variables (experimental values or "reference" constants) is collected for each of the N objects (e.g. chemical compounds). The geometrical interpretation of each object is a point in the M-dimensional space, where each variable defines an orthogonal axis. Accordingly, the data set has the form of N points in an M space. The multivariate methods seek for the structure of the data, i.e. they try to recognize systematic patterns, if present. This research area is therefore called "pattern recognition" (Kowalski and Bender, 1972; Albano *et al.*, 1978).

The various pattern recognition methods work on the basis of similarity criteria for the data points. Some of the methods are based on the concept of the Euclidean distance: the closer the points are in the M-space the more similar are the two objects. Examples of such methods, aimed mainly at classification problems, are (a) linear discriminant analysis (LDA), where the method develops a mathematical function able to separate the objects of two classes; (b) K^{th} nearest neighbour (KNN), where the classification of new objects as belonging to one class relies on the distance from the nearest objects; (c) cluster analysis, etc.

Other methods use, as similarity criterion, the fit to a unique mathematical model. They are all based on least squares procedures, and they are better suited for drug design problems as they allow the description of the data by mathematical equations, possibly implying cause–effect relationships. This paper will focus on multiple regression analysis (MRA), principal components analysis (PCA), and partial least squares analysis (PLS), pointing out the differences in the philosophy and the numerical requirements of their use.

Since all least squares methods are based on the mathematical assumptions for the analysis of variance (ANOVA), a few general requirements should be remembered to show how any analysis needs good models and good data. First, the data set under investigation is a sample of a much larger population; when it is not representative enough of its "universum" no general conclusion can be drawn outside the local range covered by the sample (Sjostrom and Wold, 1981). Second, the numerical procedure requires normalized (autoscaled) data to give to each variable the same variance, i.e. equal initial importance. If this procedure is not followed no direct comparison of the resulting statistical coefficients is possible. Then the method immediately takes away and stores the average values for each variable; they may be useful for classification purposes but they do not contain any "systematic" information. The data matrix now possibly does contain some systematic information. Each method divides it into a "relationship" (variation explained by the model) and "residuals" (unexplained variation). However, the residuals contain two types of errors: those due to experimental errors (need for good data) and those due to lack of fit (need for good models) (Deming, 1983).

While the need for good experimental data is obvious to chemists, they are aware that the state of the art in pharmacology gives biological data of poorer quality than, for instance, in physical organic chemistry. The need for good models deserves a further comment. All mathematical models are developed as the multivariate extension of Taylor expansion, i.e. the possibility of describing any mathematical function as a polynomial of n-degrees, provided the function is continuous and infinitely derivable. Accordingly, multivariate methods can be applied only to data matrices whose elements are numbers obtained, in principle, from a continuous series. Therefore, discrete variables like 1/0 to indicate the presence or absence of a substituent in a series cannot be used in this context.

Comparison of MRA, PCA and PLS

Multiple regression analysis (Draper and Smith, 1981) was developed to describe the values of a dependent variable y_i as a function of a number of independent variables x_{ia} (Eq. 1).

$$y_i = c_o + \sum_{a=1}^{A} c_a x_{ia} + \epsilon_i \qquad [1]$$

Since this method is by far the most popular multivariate approach in drug design, following the original treatment proposed by Hansch (Hansch and Leo, 1979), it is worthwhile stressing some of the implications it involves. First, MRA requires that all the "descriptor" variables are independent and error free, in order to avoid multicollinearity (which might give rise to meaningless regression coefficients), and to use the statistical tests generally reported by chemists. Second, MRA requires *a priori* knowledge that all the independent variables used in the treatment are relevant to the problem. Low regression coefficients (c_a) cannot be used to disregard one of the variables (in a data set of rate constants containing temperature as one of the variables, even if the coefficient of the "temperature" variable is low, i.e. temperature does not describe significantly the systematic variation of the set, we cannot conclude the rate constants do not depend on temperature!) Finally, MRA is insensitive to groupings of the data points; if this is the case, MRA leads to a fairly good explanation of the interclass structure, but it is unable to recognize the existence of subgroups.

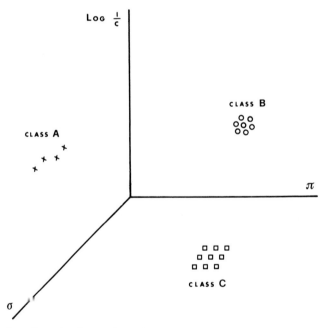

FIG. 1   A three-dimensional space formed by three variables: the biological activity (log 1/C) and two descriptors (σ and π). The data points representing the chemical compounds are grouped in three clusters (classes).

Let us consider an hypothetical example where the biological response of a series of monosubstituted compounds (log 1/C = y) is described in terms of hydrophobicity ($\pi = x_1$) and electronic effect ($\sigma = x_2$) of the substituent. Let us assume that the data points constitute three subgroups, e.g. alkyls, donors and acceptors (*vide infra*). The structure of the three-dimensional space is described in Fig. 1. The model of the MRA approach is the two-dimensional plane (two descriptor variables) illustrated in Fig. 2.

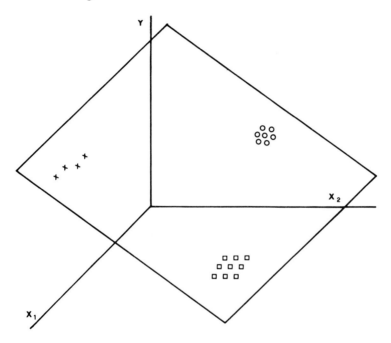

FIG. 2   The MRA solution for the data structure of Fig. 1. A unique plane is fitted to all points.

In principal components analysis (PCA) no cause–effect relation-ship is assumed, and all the M variables are treated in the same way (Mardia *et al.*, 1979). The method seeks for systematic variations in the data matrix, in order to find out the structure of the objects in the M-space. No assumption is required about the variables. The corre-lations between them are indeed used to determine the mathematical solution.

The SIMCA method, a computer package developed at the University of Umeå (Wold and Sjostrom, 1977; Albano *et al.*, 1981), is based on the philosophy of applying disjoint PC models to each class of homogenous objects. The data matrix contains elements y_{ik}, where index i is used for the experimental measurements (variables) and index k for the chemical compounds (objects). Each element is described by Eq. 2, where the number A of significant cross-terms (components) and the parameters α_i, β_{ia}, ϑ_{ak} are estimated by minimizing the squared residuals ϵ_{ik}.

$$y_{ik} = \alpha_i + \sum_{a=1}^{A} \beta_{ia} \vartheta_{ak} + \epsilon_{ik} \qquad [2]$$

In this model α_i and β_{ia} are constants which only depend upon the variables, and ϑ_{ak} depends upon the compounds. The deviations from the model are expressed by the residuals ϵ_{ik}. By autoscaling, the variables are all given the same variance, fixed to unity, in order to have the same importance in the analysis. The PCA then proceeds by model expansions to find the correct dimensionality A.

First a model with A = 0 is fitted to the data, i.e. each variable is described by its mean value α_i. After substraction of the mean values from each element y_{ik} the residuals of dimension 0 are obtained. A straight line is then fitted to these residuals, whereby the $\beta_{i1} \vartheta_{1k}$ term is estimated. Whether this first dimension is significant, i.e. whether the residuals contain systematic information, is determined by cross-validation (Wold, 1978). The new residuals for this A = 1 model are computed by subtracting the term $\beta_{i1} \vartheta_{1k}$. If the new residuals still contain systematic information additional $\beta\vartheta$ terms are subsequently estimated one after the other, until the residuals contain just noise.

For the example under examination the PCA solution is illustrated in Fig. 3; class A is described by a straight line, class B by its mean value, and class C by a plane. Clearly this solution represents the data structure much better than that obtained by MRA. Consequently, the prediction of new data is much better, provided the new compound can be easily classified as belonging to one of the groups. However, it should be stressed that no cause–effect relationship is assumed in PCA. Philosophically speaking, we just compare three experimental measurements: the biological activity and the octanol/water partition coefficients of our series and the ionization constants of benzoic acids. Accordingly, any explanation of why a chemical compound has a certain biological activity is not straightforward.

When the main objective of the data analysis is prediction rather than interpretation the mathematical model can be refined to give a better fit of the data points. With autoscaling all variables have equal initial importance, and this is relevant for interpretation. A refined model can be obtained by reweighting the variables, i.e. by multiplying each variable by its modelling power ψ_i, defined in Eq. 3. Here s_i and s_{iy} are the residual standard deviations for variable i with A significant components and with A = 0, respectively. This means that variables for which the $\beta\vartheta$ terms contain little or no information will have modelling powers close to zero. Thus, with this type of reweighting, such variables are given small weights.

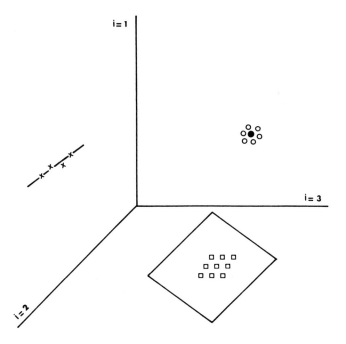

FIG. 3   The PCA solution obtained by the SIMCA method for the data structure of Fig. 1. Each class is fitted by a disjoint PC model

$$\psi_i = 1 - \frac{s_i}{s_{iy}}$$ [3]

However, a method able to cope both with prediction and interpretation is highly desirable in drug design and, in general, in bioorganic chemistry. In other words, a statistical approach allowing the prediction of activities with the best possible precision and relating these activities to structural parameters such as electronic demand, hydrophobicity, steric requirements, etc. is highly suited for this topic area.

This is now accomplished by the recently developed method called partial least squares analysis (PLS) (Albano *et al.*, 1981; Wold, 1977; Wold *et al.*, 1980; Wold, 1981). Also in this case a dependent variable y (the biological response) is described in terms of a number of explanatory variables x_a (the descriptors σ, π, E_s, etc.). However, no assumption on the relevance of individual variables is required. The method works out the principal components for the descriptors block (Eq. 4) and then seeks for a simple linear relationship between these components and the biological response (Eq. 5).

$$x_{ik} = \alpha_i + \sum_{a=1}^{A} \beta_{ia}\xi_{ak} + \epsilon_{ik} \qquad [4]$$

$$y_k = \bar{y} + \sum_{a=1}^{A} \varrho_a\xi_{ak} + \epsilon_k \qquad [5]$$

Assume that, in our example, the activity depends upon a certain blend of electronic and solubility requirements. PLS first finds the relationships between them (Fig. 4a) by PCA, and then that between the new component ξ and the biological response y by ordinary regression methods (Fig.4b). If the linear relationship between the explanatory variables is pretty good, one single component, and therefore one single effect, may be sufficient to explain the biological response. However, this unique "true" effect can be explained as a linear combination of our "reference" descriptors.

If the descriptor variables are not highly correlated the number of components could be as many as the number of variables. In this case

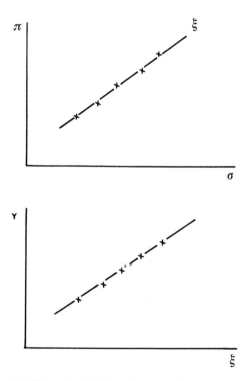

FIG. 4   Illustration of the PLS method: (a) The PC solution is found for the descriptor variables; (b) a relationship is tested between the dependent variable and the first principal component.

the numerical solution obtained in PLS is the same as in MRA. The experience available shows, however, that the number of components required is usually much less than the number of variables. Moreover, PLS is able to spot the existence of subgroups. For the example in Fig. 1 one should have three different PLS models for each of the subgroup.

Instead of this two-step procedure (PCA + MRA) it is possible to make a single analysis accomplishing the two steps simultaneously, by means of an appropriate algorithm illustrated in detail in Albano *et al.* (1981). This algorithm is indeed used in the SIMCA/PLS package, which also contains the PLS2 method, already used in medicinal chemistry (Hellberg *et al.*, 1982).

This latter method applies when there are a number of dependent variables. The problem is therefore defined by a dependent matrix Y and an independent matrix X. The question is whether it is possible to describe the elements of the Y matrix as a simple function of the elements of the X matrix. In principle such a problem is solved by computing a PC model for each of the two matrices and then looking for linear relationships between the principal components of the two blocks. Again in SIMCA the two steps are accomplished simultaneously (Albano *et al.*, 1981). The PLS2 analysis results therefore in a description of the X matrix by one PC-like model (Eq. 4), a description of the Y matrix by another PC-like model (Eq. 6), and predictive relations between the latent variables ξ and η (Eq. 7).

$$Y_{jk} = \alpha_j + \sum_{a=1}^{A} \beta_{ja} \eta_{ak} + \epsilon_{jk} \tag{6}$$

$$\eta_{ak} = \varrho_a \xi_{ak} + \epsilon_k \tag{7}$$

Suppose we have for our example series three biological responses (e.g. toxicity, a prefixed response, and an effective dose) and we want to describe them in terms of σ, π, and E_s. These quantities define a Y space (Fig. 5a) and an X space (Fig. 5b). The PLS2 solution is obtained in such a way to maximize the relationship between the two blocks.

Also PLS2 is sensitive to groupings. When the data structure exhibits the presence of subgroups, disjoint PLS2 models should be used for each group.

Discussion

The implications of applying multivariate statistical methods in describing biological activities of chemical compounds, and therefore in drug design, deserves a further comment. In particular some of the

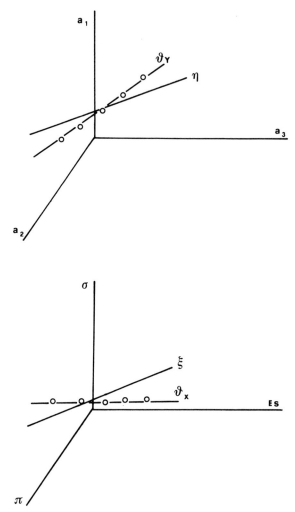

FIG. 5   Illustration of the PLS2 method. The dependent variables y (activities) and the independent variables x (descriptors) define two different spaces. The PCA solution of both them is found under the constraint that the latent variables of the X space (ξ) should be linearly related to the latent variables of the Y space (η).

limitations induced by the special features of biological data should be stressed.

It is intuitive that the chemical structure of a drug must have some well defined characteristics to be able to interact with the receptor site. According to Hansch (Hansch and Leo, 1979) the level of biological activity can be a regular and well behaved function of structurally related parameters. However, any drastic change in structure may result in a discontinuity of the structure–activity relationship and inactivity will result (Dunn and Wold, 1980a). The reasons for this discontinuity can be diverse, since any type of structural change that inhibits the appropriate interaction with the receptor site will lead to inactivity.

As a consequence the structure of a data set including active and inactive compounds is usually asymmetric (Dunn and Wold, 1980a) (Fig. 6), i.e. the active compounds have structure while the inactive ones have no structure and are spread all around.

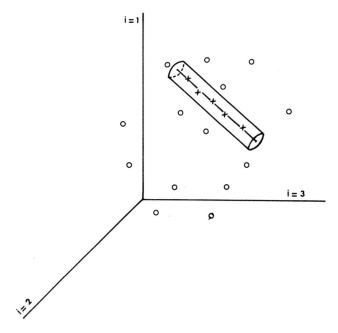

FIG. 6   Asymmetric data structure. The active compounds are modelled by a straight line, while the inactive compounds cannot be modelled.

Clearly in such asymmetric cases none of the statistical methods aimed at classification (LDA, KNN, etc.) can work. No mathematical function can be described to divide the active from the inactive compounds. Nor can MRA describe properly the whole data set. On the contrary, PCA is a suitable approach to describe these cases, since a mathematical model can be fitted to the active compounds, while the inactive ones cannot be modelled. Accordingly, a compound will be classified as active or not depending upon its position within or outside the confidence region around the "active" model.

A further limitation with MRA in describing biological activities is its insensitivity to groupings in the data points. MRA is unable to recognize the existence of subgroups in the data. Consequently, MRA will describe fairly well the intergroup structure, but it cannot describe the intragroup structure.

For the example described in Fig. 2, where the data points are grouped in three bunches in the data space, MRA implying *a priori* to fit a plane to the data, will find the best plane fitting the three bunches, irrespectively of how the points behave within each group. The statistical tests are all right, but this is because it is not realized that groupings dramatically change the number of degrees of freedom. This is probably the reason why most of the Hansch treatments by MRA in QSAR do give fairly good results (correlation coefficients ca. 0.9): the plane is fitted just to a few clusters. It should be realized that, besides the philosophical requirements of knowing *a priori* the relevance of descriptors, whenever the data points are grouped, MRA cannot give results better than these. On the contrary, PCA, which has the same mathematical form as MRA, by applying disjoint models for each group, can give a much better description, and therefore prediction, of the biological activities.

Such groupings were already observed studying the substituent effects in reactivity (Alunni *et al.*, 1983) and spectral data (Johnels *et al.*, 1983). There is no reason to doubt that a similar situation applies also to biological data. Such a study is at present under investigation (Codarin *et al.*, 1983) and its results will be reported elsewhere.

Since PCA does not involve a cause−effect relationship the state of the art of chemometrics in QSAR applications to drug design seems to indicate PLS (and PLS2) as the most promising approaches. PCA can still be successfully used to investigate bioorganic mechanisms or the information content of biological tests. However, the description and prediction of activity as a function of well defined "descriptors", in line with the Hansch approach, is handled by PLS better than by PCA or MRA. Indeed PLS does not require the restrictions needed in MRA and has all the same advantages as PCA, such as the sensitivity to groupings, the possibility of excluding irrelevant variables, etc.

The application of PLS in medicinal chemistry is in its early stages. The first such work (Hellberg *et al.*, 1982) has shown that a number of structural descriptors can be used to classify beta-adrenergic compounds as agonists or antagonists, and to predict their biological activity. Furthermore PLS can handle asymmetric cases and disjoint groups. However, it might be that the descriptors presently used (σ, π, E_s, etc.), mainly derived from physical organic chemistry, are not suitable enough to rationalize the behaviour of compounds in a complex environment such as *in vivo*. The use of more appropriate descriptors directly derived from biological data (Codarin *et al.*, 1983) can greatly improve the usefulness of these modelling methods.

Example

The SIMCA/PLS method was applied in our laboratory to a data set regarding the antitumor activities of 13 para-substituted aryldimethyl-triazenes, measured at the University of Trieste (Lassiani *et al.*, 1983). They include toxicity (test 1), the molar dose which produces a predetermined effect on the primary tumour (test 2) and on the weight (test 3) and number (test 4) of metastases, together with the effect produced by the maximum non toxic dose in the same experiments, in terms of treated over control ratios (tests 5–7). These data were analysed together with a few literature series on the same compounds (Lassiani *et al.*, in preparation; Linda *et al.*, in preparation).

The data set raised a number of problems: (a) the information content of the various tests; (b) the description of activities by models able to predict new data; (c) the statistical base to show whether these compounds exhibit specific antimetastatic activity.

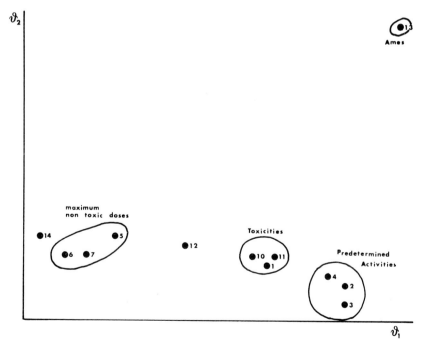

FIG. 7   Plot of the first against the second component for the experimental measurements of antitumour activities.

The data set was investigated under a variety of conditions. Considering the substituents as variables and the biological tests as objects, PCA makes it possible to determine the relative information content of the individual tests. The results of this analysis are illustrated in Fig. 7. Only the Ames test, which refers to mutageneticity, is not systematic with the others. Excluding this, PCA is able to explain over 90% of the total variation with a single component, i.e. all tests lie fairly well on a straight line. However, along this first principal component, one can recognize subgroups of objects which indeed define toxicities, predetermined activities, and effective doses (Lassiani *et al.*, in preparation).

On transposing the matrix, i.e. considering the substituted triazenes as objects and the activities as variables, three components are needed to explain up to 70% of the total variance. The three plots illustrated in Figs 8 – 10 show the grouping of substituents in the space defined by the principal components. This grouping stresses again the hazard of using MRA, which can only describe the interclass structure. Again, the $\beta_1\beta_2$ plot, which indicates the relationships between the variables, shows the differences between the various types of activities (Fig. 11).

Clearly the PCA shows that, while the predetermined activities all lie within a small area and therefore are unable to give evidence of any difference between the decrease of the primary tumour and that of metastases, by using the T/C ratios the influence on the primary tumour

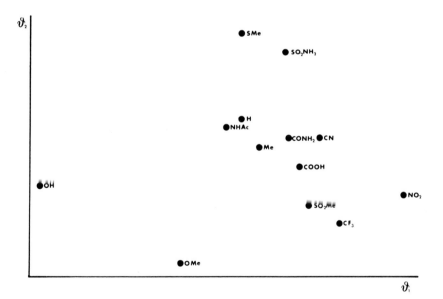

FIG. 8   Plot of the first against the second component for the para substituted aryldimethyl-triazenes.

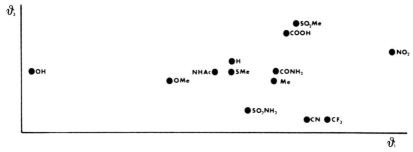

FIG. 9   Plot of the first against the third component for the para substituted aryldimethyltriazenes.

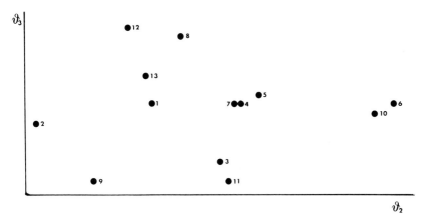

FIG. 10   Plot of the second against the third component for the para substituted aryldimethyl-triazenes. Numbers identify substituents as follows: 1 = OH, 2 = OMe, 3 = Me, 4 = NHAc, 5 = H, 6 = SMe, 7 = CONH$_2$, 8 = COOH, 9 = CF$_3$, 10 = SO$_2$NH$_2$, 11 = CN, 12 = SO$_2$Me, 13 = NO$_2$.

is almost opposite to that on metastases. The selective antimetastatic properties of these compounds, which cannot be seen by MRA or by activities at a predetermined level can therefore be stated (Lassiani *et al.*, in preparation).

The subsequent step of the analysis is to model these activities in terms of the usual descriptors. We considered σ and σ^+ for electronic demand, log P, its square and π for hydrophobicity, MR for polarizability, the E$_s$ and the Verloop parameters for the steric requirements. The block of activities (Y block: 11 activities) was modelled by the block of descriptors (X block: 12 descriptors) by the PLS2 method.

The results of this analysis are quite interesting. Two components are significant, which means that two distinct effects can be transported from the descriptors to the activities. The variables defining the first component are mainly of the electronic and steric type, whereas the variables relevant for the second component are those describing

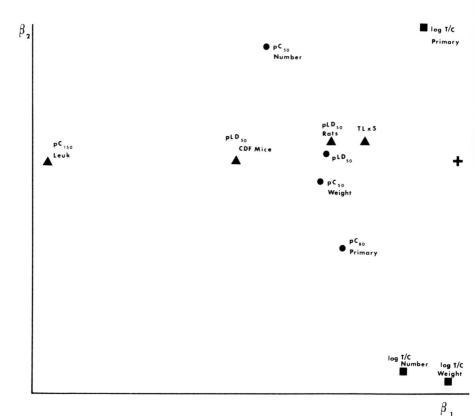

FIG. 11   Relationship between the antitumour activities measured on para substituted aryl-dimethyltriazenes.

hydrophibicity and polarizability. The fraction of variance of the Y-block described by the two components is 46%. Since the total structure of the Y-block described by PCA was 72% for A = 3, it can be concluded that these descriptors are able to explain up to two thirds of the systematic variation of the experimental activity data.

However, the data set is not homogeneous, as illustrated by the plots reported in Figs 12 and 13. Figure 12 shows the diagram of the first latent variable of the $X(\xi_1)$ against the $Y(\eta_1)$ block: there is a clear separation of substituents according to their electronic effects. Analogously, Fig. 13 shows the diagram of the second latent variables: again a strong grouping is evident, on the basis of the hydrophobic properties.

The data points are therefore grouped in the Y-space, as already seen by PCA in Figs 8–10. Unfortunately, the number of available points is too small to attempt a better description on disjoint groups.

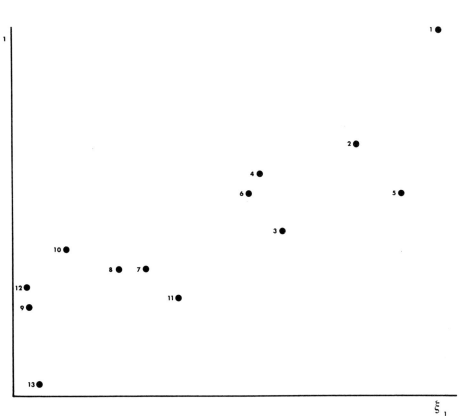

FIG. 12 Plot of the first component of the descriptors block against the first component of the variables block. Numbers identify the substituents as in Fig. 10.

Further information obtained by the PLS2 analysis is given by the relationship between the variables, considering both activities and descriptors. These are illustrated by the β_1 versus β_2 plot reported in Fig. 14. The predetermined activities are directly related to E_s and inversely related to the electronic parameters, whereas the maximum non-toxic doses are more strictly related to the hydrophobic parameters.

The interpretation of this plot will require further investigation. The final step of this analysis should have been the PLS analysis for each individual activity measurement. However, once more the PLS analysis cannot give satisfactory results on the whole set of substituents because of the existing groupings, and the number of available objects is too small to operate on disjoint groups.

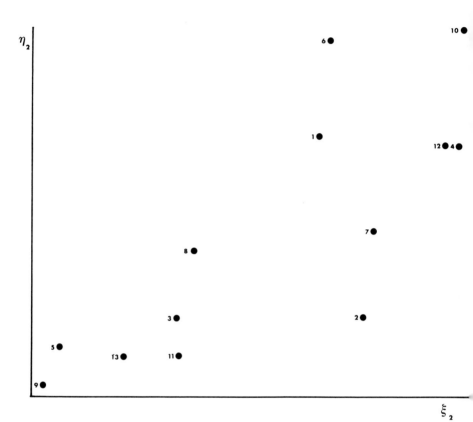

FIG. 13   Plot of the second component of the descriptors block against the second component of the variables block. Numbers identify substituents as in Fig. 10.

Acknowledgements

The author wishes to express his thanks to S. Wold and his group in Umeå for providing the SIMCA/PLS package and for encouragement and helpful discussion, to S. Alunni and G. Giulietti (Perugia) for their valuable cooperation, to L. Lassiani and C. Nisi (Trieste) for providing data prior to their publication, and to P. Linda and F. Rubessa (Trieste) for discussion.

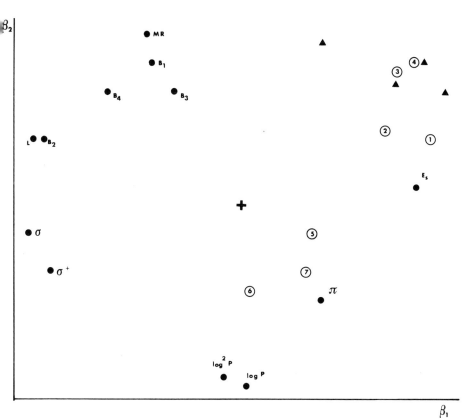

FIG. 14 Relationship between the variables in the PLS2 analysis. Variables near to each other or opposite with respect to the centre of the diagram are highly correlated.

References

Albano, C., Dunn, W.J., Edlund, U., Johansson, E., Norden, B., Sjostrom, M. and Wold, S. (1978). *Anal. Chim. Acta* **103**, 429–443.

Albano, C., Blomquist, G., Coomans, D., Dunn, W.J., Edlund, U., Eliasson, B., Hellberg, S., Johansson, E., Norden, B., Sjostrom, M., Soderstrom, B., Wold, H. and Wold, S. (1981). *In* "Symposium i anvent statistik" (A. Hoskuldsen *et al.*, eds), pp. 183–218. NEUCC, RECAU and RECKU, Kopenhamn.

Alunni, S., Clementi, S., Edlund, U., Johnels, D., Hellberg, S., Sjostrom, M. and Wold, S. (1983). *Acta Chem. Scand.* **B37**, 47–53.

Box, G.E.P., Hunter, W.G. and Hunter, J.S. (1978). "Statistics for Experimenters", Wiley, New York.

Codarin, M., Linda, P., Lassiani, L., Rubessa, F., Alunni, S., Clementi, S., Sjostrom, M., Wold, S. and Dunn, W.J. (1983). Submitted to *J. Med. Chem.*

Deming, S. (1983). *Anal. Chim. Acta* **150/1**, 183–198.

Draper, N. and Smith, M. (1981). "Applied Regression Analysis", 2nd ed., Wiley-Interscience, New York.

Dunn, W.J. and Wold, S. (1978a). *Acta Chem. Scand.* **B32**, 536–542.
Dunn, W.J. and Wold, S. (1978b). *J. Med. Chem.* **21**, 1001–1007.
Dunn, W.J. and Wold, S. (1980a). *J. Med. Chem.* **23**, 595–599.
Dunn, W.J. and Wold, S. (1980b). *Bioorg. Chem.* **9**, 505–523.
Dunn, W.J. and Wold, S. (1981). *Bioorg. Chem.* **10**, 29–45.
Dunn, W.J., Wold, S. and Martin, Y.C. (1978). *J. Med. Chem.* **21**, 922–930.
Hansch, C. and Leo, A. (1979). "Substituent Constants for Correlation Analysis in Chemistry and Biology", Wiley-Interscience, New York.
Hellberg, S., Wold, S. and Dunn, W.J. (1982). Submitted to *J. Chem. Inf. Comput. Sci.*
Johnels, D., Clementi, S., Dunn, W.J., Edlund, U., Grahn, H., Hellberg, S., Sjostrom, M. and Wold, S. (1983). *J. Chem. Soc., Perkin Trans.* **2**, 863–871.
Kowalski, B.R. and Bender, C.F. (1972). *J. Am. Chem. Soc.* **94**, 5632–5639.
Lassiani, L., Nisi, C., Sava, G., Girardi, T. and Cuman, R. (1983). Submitted to *Quant. Struct.–Act. Relat.*
Lassiani, L., Nisi, C., Rubessa, F., Codarin, M., Linda, P., Alunni, S. and Clementi, S. Principal components analysis of antitumour tests, in preparation.
Linda, P., Lassiani, L., Nisi, C., Rubessa, F., Alunni, S., Clementi, S., Dunn, W.J., Sjostrom, M. and Wold, S. Partial least squares analysis of the antitumour activity of aryldimethyltriazenes, in preparation.
Mardia, K.V., Kent, J.T. and Bibby, J.M. (1979). "Multivariate Analysis", Academic Press, London.
Massart, D.L., Dijkstra, A. and Kaufman, L. (1978). "Evaluation and Optimization of Laboratory Methods and Analytical Procedures". Elsevier, Amsterdam.
Sjostrom, M. and Wold, S. (1981). *Acta Chem. Scand.* **B35**, 537–554.
Wold, H. (1977). *In* "Mathematical Economics and Game Theory. Essays in Honour of Oscar Morgestern" (R. Hern and O. Moeschlin, eds). Springer-Verlag, Berlin.
Wold, H. (1981). "Systems under Indirect Observation: Causality–Structure–Prediction" (K.G. Joreskog and H. Wold, eds), Vol. 2. North-Holland, Amsterdam.
Wold, H. (1983). *In* "Proceedings of the IUFoST Symposium on Food Chemistry and Data Analysis". Oslo 1982, Applied Science Pub., London.
Wold, S. (1978). *Technometrics* **20**, 397–406.
Wold, S. and Sjostrom, M. (1977). *In* "Chemometrics: Theory and Application" (B.R. Kowalski, ed.), ACS Symp. Series n. 52, 243–282. American Chemical Society, Washington.
Wold, S., Wold, H., Dunn, W.J. and Ruhe, A. (1980). The collinearity problem in linear and non linear regression: the partial least squares approach to generalized inverses, Report UMINF 83.80, ISSN 0348-0542. Umeå University, Insts. of information processing and chemistry.

Discussion

Chairman: Professor Tomlinson

Dr Choplin

There are two parts in this type of study: the data analysis, and the preparation of the data. The representation of molecules by matrices is really the key problem. I regret you did not emphasize this problem.

Professor Clementi
My main interest was, from an empirical point of view, applying correct statistical procedure in the best possible way on available experiment measurements. The other point is relevant but I am not competent enough to discuss it.

Professor Tomlinson
I saw very exciting techniques here for the interpretation and understanding of existing data – but how will your technique lead to the designing of new drugs? Will it generate any new compound?

Professor Clementi
Provided that the activity set can be described in terms of the usual descriptors that can be found in the literature, using the mathematical model that has been developed, the activity of any possible new compounds can easily be predicted.

Professor Tomlinson
It is a pure extrapolation procedure?

Professor Clementi
Provided that we stay fairly near to the local range where the mathematical equation has been developed, this procedure is simply a local linearization of what are probably very complex problems, so that the linear model holds only very near the region where it has been developed.

Professor Tomlinson
But with that system can we still talk in terms of spanned substituent space and unspanned substituent space, as Professor Hansch has often propounded?

Professor Clementi
I prefer to look at the mathematical model to see whether a structure can be found in our data set. After doing that, if there is a structure, we can get a good prediction.

Professor Hansch
Let us say that you were treating data in which only π and σ are important and thus you have different sets of structure–activity relationship data. Going from one set of biological activities to another, a new vector, a new combination of π and σ is constantly being created. It seems to me that one of the big disadvantages of this is that it provides no feeling of how π and σ will behave.

I am not sure that even if it is related back, like in the partial least squares fit, it may help. It seems to be a very significant disadvantage of this approach. Looking at sets of chemicals, one begins to see certain patterns about how hydrophobic effects behave, and how electronic effects behave. I would rather take a poor mathematical description of the data, but keep this picture of how the different effects are working for its value in relating one kind of activity to another.

Professor Clementi

First, it was just a simple example. However, if there are quite a number of activity measurements of the same kind (like in physical organic chemistry, we have a number of measurements for electrophilic substitution, for nucleophilic substitution and so on), statistical parameters can be obtained with a chemical meaning or can at least be related to certain chemical meanings, which are able to describe the activity set better than multiple regression can.

6 Pattern Recognition as a Tool for Drug Design

S. WOLD*, W.J. DUNN III[+] and S. HELLBERG*

*Research Group for Chemometrics, Umeå
University, S-901 87 Umeå, Sweden*

[+]*Department of Medicinal Chemistry and
Pharmacognosy, College of Pharmacy,
University of Illinois, PO Box 6998, Chicago,
Illinois 60680, USA*

Introduction

Pattern recognition (PARC) is a battery of data analytical methods which have been terribly misused in drug design and related areas. The results of a recent evaluation of the area indicate that, because basic statistical conditions are not fulfilled, more than 50% of the published applications of PARC in QSAR are fortuitous chance correlations (Wold *et al.*, 1982; Wold and Dunn, 1983).

It is therefore natural that the application of PARC in drug design is seen with some scepticism, as being perhaps more fantasy than fact. However, the character of the problems in drug design and QSAR is such that PARC is often the natural choice of method for the data analysis. Hence, there is a need for the separation of fact from fantasy in the field.

In fact, the theory and underlying concepts of PARC are easy to understand and master because they are closely related to the ordinary experimental approach of chemistry and pharmacology. Provided that some simple rules of statistics and chemistry are obeyed, PARC works

DRUG DESIGN: FACT OR FANTASY
ISBN 0.12.388180.3

well. This we shall try to show in the present article, using as illustration a QSAR application of the SIMCA method.

What is Pattern Recognition (PARC)?

The primary objective of PARC is to produce rules for classifying objects (here compounds) into one of a number of given classes. These rules are derived from compounds "known" to belong to either of the classes (the training set) and multivariate data, X, characterizing these compounds (see Fig. 1).

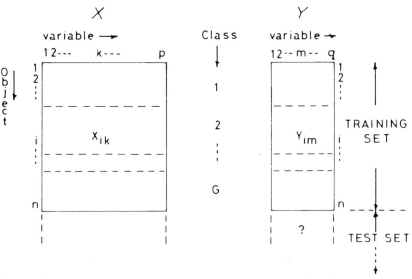

FIG. 1   The data in the generalized pattern recognition problem are organized in one or two tables, matrices. The matrix X contains "independent" variables characterizing the structure of the compounds such as sigma, pi, molecular refractivity, etc.

On PARC 3 and 4, there is also a matrix of "dependent" variables with one or several columns. In drug design and QSAR, these variables describe the biological activity of the compounds.

The data X (and Y) are divided into two sets: (A) The training set, used to develop the typical "data pattern" of the classes 1 to G and (B) the test set containing compounds of unknown class and on levels 3 and 4, with unknown Y-values.

The first phase of PARC, the "training phase" is analogous to the chemical practice of "learning" the regularities of classes of compounds from model compounds representative of the classes.

In a second phase of PARC, the derived rules are used to classify new, unassigned, compounds (the test set). This is done by applying the rules to the multidimensional data characterizing these new compounds.

On higher ambition levels of PARC, levels 3 and 4 (Albano *et al.*, 1978), one also wishes to model and predict dependent variables (Y) in some or all of the classes. On level 3, there is one single y-variable, while on level 4 there are several y-variables. In drug design and QSAR, Y usually consists of quantitative measures of the biological activity of the investigated compounds.

Hence, in PARC 3 and 4, the training phase also consists of the development of quantitative models for predicting the dependent variables Y from the characterizing variables X (Fig. 1).

We can see PARC 3 and 4 as a problem of multivariable calibration. We wish to develop calibrated models that allow us to use multivariate data, X (here structure descriptors), to predict one or several dependent variables, Y. To accomplish this, we have a training set of compounds for which both X and Y are given and for which we "know" the class they belong to.

Once the calibrated models are developed by the use of the training set, the models can be used together with X-data to classify new compounds to one of the given classes or as a member of none of them (an outlier). In addition, the X-data can be used to predict the values of the dependent variables for an object that is classified as belonging to a class for which a model of Y has been developed.

Example

Mukherjee *et al.* (1976) measured the beta-adrenergic activity for 37 substituted phenethyl-amines (Fig. 2). Seventeen of these were clear antagonists (class 1) and 15 were agonists (class 2). For the antagonists, the binding constant to a purified receptor (y_1) and the relative antagonist activity against stimulation of beta-adrenergic coupled adenyl cyclase (y_2) were reported. For the agonists, the same binding constant, the agonist activity and the intrinsic activity (y_3) were reported. Of the compounds, five had weak or no activity and were used as a test set. Below we describe how the structural variation between the 37 compounds was translated to nine variables related to properties of the substituents R1, R2, X and Y (Fig. 2).

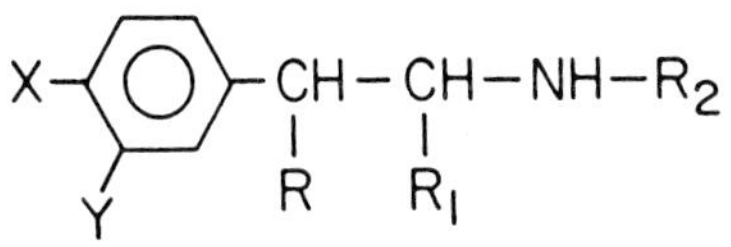

FIG. 2   In the example, the data concern 37 compounds of the above structure. For the data, see Table 1.

TABLE 1a

Data in the example. For X, see 1b.

OBJ.	X	Y	R	R(1)	R(2)	CLASS	ACT.Y1.	pkB.Y2.	IA.Y3.
1	18	18	OH	2	1	2	4.39	4.55	0.87
2	18	18	OH	3	1	2	4.42	4.74	0.71
3	18	18	OH	1	2	2	5.00	5.07	0.75
4	18	18	OH	1	4	2	5.85	5.77	1.00
5	18	18	OH	3	4	2	4.35	4.62	0.72
6	18	18	OH	3	5	2	4.51	4.41	0.64
7	18	18	OH	1	6	2	6.33	6.17	1.10
8	18	18	OH	1	7	2	6.37	6.17	1.10
9	18	18	H	1	8	2	4.68	4.33	0.25
10	18	18	H	1	9	2	5.04	4.62	0.25
11	18	18	OH	1	10	2	7.10	7.22	1.20
12	18	18	H	1	11	2	5.04	4.64	0.17
13	18	19	OH	1	4	2	6.00	5.62	0.28
14	18	19	OH	1	4	2	5.48	6.19	0.24
15	18	19	OH	1	12	2	7.10	7.85	0.27
16	17	20	OH	1	1	1	3.51	4.08	
17	17	19	OH	1	2	1	3.66	4.19	
18	17	18	OH	1	2	1	3.87	4.28	
19	17	18	OH	1	3	1	4.29	4.66	
20	20	18	OH	1	4	1	5.89	5.38	
21	18	17	OH	1	4	1	4.96	4.82	
22	17	18	OH	2	1	1	4.52	4.46	
23	20	20	OH	1	4	1	6.40	6.24	
24	19	17	OH	1	4	1	5.80	5.89	
25	17	17	OH	16	1	1	3.85	4.29	
26	17	17	OH	2	2	1	4.07	5.04	
27	21	17	OH	3	4	1	5.35	4.85	
28	18	17	OH	2	8	1	5.74	5.06	
29	18	17	OH	2	13	1	6.62	5.85	
30	18	17	OH	2	14	1	6.89	6.74	
31	18	22	OH	2	13	1	7.22	7.12	
32	17	23	OH	2	15	1	5.64	5.11	
33	18	18	OH	1	1	0	4.04	<3.70	
34	18	17	OH	1	1	0	<3.00	<3.70	
35	18	17	H	1	1	0	<3.00	<3.70	
36	18	18	H	1	1	0	<3.00	<3.70	
37	17	17	H	1	1	0	<3.00	<3.70	

Substituents X, Y, R(1) and R(2) are displayed in Tables 1c and 1d.

TABLE 1b

The table X of the example.

OBJ.	x-1 pKa	x-2 fph	x-3 fR1	x-4 fR2	x-5 sigmaR2	x-6 EsR2	x-7 sigma-p	x-8 B-4	x-9 L
1	8.93	1.14	0.70	0.19	0.49	1.24	− 0.37	2.74	1.93
2	8.93	1.14	1.23	0.19	0.49	1.24	− 0.37	2.74	1.93
3	9.29	1.14	0.19	0.70	0.00	0.00	− 0.37	2.74	1.93
4	9.90	1.14	0.19	1.64	− 0.10	− 0.47	− 0.37	2.74	1.93
5	9.90	1.14	1.23	1.64	− 0.10	− 0.47	− 0.37	2.74	1.93
6	9.93	1.14	1.23	2.35	− 0.20	− 0.51	− 0.37	2.74	1.93
7	9.19	1.14	0.19	2.83	− 0.13	− 0.93	− 0.37	2.74	1.93
8	9.19	1.14	0.19	2.56	− 0.13	− 0.93	− 0.37	2.74	1.93
9	10.03	1.14	0.19	2.42	− 0.08	− 0.38	− 0.37	2.74	1.93
10	10.29	1.14	0.19	3.36	− 0.13	− 0.93	− 0.37	2.74	1.93
11	9.29	1.14	0.19	2.43	− 0.30	− 1.60	− 0.37	2.74	1.93
12	10.22	1.14	0.19	2.95	− 0.08	− 0.38	− 0.37	2.74	1.93
13	9.94	− 0.07	0.19	1.64	− 0.19	− 0.47	− 0.37	2.74	1.93
14	9.77	− 0.07	0.19	1.64	− 0.19	− 0.47	− 0.37	2.74	1.93
15	9.29	− 0.07	0.19	3.80	− 0.30	− 1.60	− 0.37	2.74	1.93
16	8.93	2.66	0.19	0.19	0.49	1.24	0.00	2.00	1.00
17	9.29	0.55	0.19	0.70	0.00	0.00	0.00	2.00	1.00
18	9.29	1.36	0.19	0.70	0.00	0.00	0.00	2.00	1.00
19	9.61	1.36	0.19	1.23	− 0.10	0.07	0.00	2.00	1.00
20	9.90	2.04	0.19	1.64	− 0.19	− 0.47	0.23	1.80	3.52
21	9.90	1.36	0.19	1.64	− 0.19	− 0.47	− 0.37	2.74	1.93
22	8.93	1.36	0.70	0.19	0.49	1.24	0.00	2.00	1.00
23	9.90	3.34	0.19	1.64	− 0.19	− 0.47	0.23	1.80	3.52
24	9.90	0.55	0.19	1.64	− 0.19	− 0.47	0.03	3.08	4.06
25	8.46	1.90	0.02	0.19	0.49	1.24	0.00	2.00	1.00
26	9.29	1.90	0.70	0.70	0.00	0.00	0.00	2.00	1.00
27	9.90	− 0.94	1.23	1.64	− 0.19	− 0.47	0.28	3.48	5.50
28	9.03	1.36	0.70	2.42	− 0.08	− 0.38	− 0.37	2.74	1.93
29	8.16	1.36	0.70	2.77	− 0.13	− 0.93	− 0.37	2.74	1.93
30	9.29	1.36	0.70	3.90	− 0.13	− 0.93	− 0.37	2.74	1.93
31	8.16	1.04	0.70	2.77	− 0.13	− 0.93	− 0.37	2.74	1.93
32	10.26	1.96	0.70	2.24	− 0.30	− 1.60	0.00	2.00	1.00
33	8.93	1.14	0.19	0.19	0.49	1.24	− 0.37	2.74	1.93
34	8.93	1.36	0.19	0.19	0.49	1.24	− 0.37	2.74	1.93
35	8.93	1.36	0.19	0.19	0.49	1.24	− 0.37	2.74	1.93
36	8.93	1.14	0.19	0.19	0.49	1.24	− 0.37	2.74	1.93
37	9.80	1.90	0.19	0.19	0.49	1.24	0.00	2.00	1.00

TABLE 1c

Substituents R_1 and R_2.

No.	Formula
1	H
2	CH_3
3	C_2H_5
4	$CH(CH_3)_2$
5	$CH(CH_2CH_2)_2$
6	$CH(CH_3)CH_2C_6H_4\text{-}4\text{-}OH$
7	$CH(CH_3)CH_2C_6H_3\text{-}3,4\text{-}OCH_2O$
8	$CH_2CH_2C_6H_4\text{-}4\text{-}OH$
9	$CH(CH_3)(CH_2)_2C_6H_4\text{-}4\text{-}OH$
10	$C(CH_3)_2CH_2C_6H_4\text{-}4\text{-}OH$
11	$(CH_2)_3C_6H_4\text{-}4\text{-}OH$
12	$C(CH_3)_2CH_2C_6H_5$
13	$CH(CH_3)CH_2OC_6H_5$
14	$CH(CH_3(CH_2)_2C_6H_5$
15	$C(CH_3)_3$
16	CH_2CH_2OH

TABLE 1d

Substituents X and Y

No.	Formula
17	H
18	OH
19	$NHSO_2CH_3$
20	Cl
21	$CH_2SO_2NH_2$
22	$CH_2SO_2N(CH_3)_2$
23	OCH_3

Problem Formulation

The reformulation of the original drug design problem to one that can be analysed by PARC, i.e. the selection of classes, compounds, biological measurements and structure descriptor variables, is the most important and most difficult part of the PARC. Hence, this part is rarely discussed and never taught. We shall adhere to this tradition and assume that the drug designer understands his problem so well that the classes can be selected to consist of pharmacologically and chemically similar compounds.

The similarity condition is related to the mathematical and philosophical fact that all empirical models, including those being the basis of PARC and multiple regression (MR), are in one way or another linearizations of complicated functions. Since linearizations are valid only in limited intervals, the data they are to approximate must be measured on processes with a limited variation.

In chemistry and pharmacology, this corresponds to the fact that empirical models can be developed for series of similar compounds, but rarely for sets of structurally diverse compounds.

Often one tries to handle active and inactive compounds as two classes. One should then be aware that the set of inactive classes often does not constitute a proper homogeneous class. The inactives may be inactive due to the lack of any of many essential features for activity. This leads to the so called asymmetric problem (Dunn and Wold, 1980a and b) where only one of the classes can be modelled.

In the example we have two natural classes, antagonists and agonists. There is no information about possible chemical or pharmacological subgroups inside these classes.

Compounds
The second part of the problem formulation is to find representative compounds for each class. This is the problem of experimental design that is similar in all investigations; how to spread the costly "experiments" over the accessible domain in an optimal way, see e.g. Box *et al.* (1978). Just one example of a bad design with four possible substituents at four sites (1121 denotes substituents no 1 at sites 1, 2 and 4 and substituents 2 at site 3): 1111, 2111, 3111, 4111, 1211, 1311, 1411, 1121, 1131, 1141, 1112, 1113, 1114. This "design" (rather lack of) is bad because one site is varied at a time. Thus no information about the joint influence of the sites on the activity is obtained. Instead a set like 1111, 2222, 3333, 4444, 1234, 2341, 3412, 4123, 3142, 4213, 1324 and 2431 provides a much better representation.

The simple rule is that in multivariate problems, the compounds must be selected so that all structural features that vary should be varied simultaneously, not one at a time.

Biological measurements
This is of course the most crucial question, where only a few generalities can be made. The biological measurements must map the final purpose of the drug. This is difficult to achieve with one single measurement and therefore several biological effect variables are often necessary.

Surprisingly, the PARC 4 problem with several dependent y-variables is numerically and statistically more stable than PARC 3 or PARC 2 problems with one or no y-variables. Hence, one can strongly recommend the inclusion of as many *relevant* measurements of the biological effect of a drug as possible. This increases the amount of information in the data and makes the data analysis simpler.

How to translate chemical structure to numbers
The specification of the descriptor data X is essential in PARC. These data must be related to the classification problem and in PARC 3 and 4 also to the levels of the data Y. It is surprising that in published PARC QSAR papers, the principle of the selection of X seems more to be the ease of making this automatically by a computer than the chemical and pharmacological relevance of X. This has lead to the widespread use of one–zero variables describing the occurrence–nonoccurrence of structural fragments in the investigated compounds. However, the success is not convincing; only one valid application based on fragment occurrences has been published according to the evaluation of Wold *et al.* (1982). Redl *et al.* (1974) also have negative experiences of the approach. Furthermore, the fragment occurrence variables do not have the right continuity properties for PARC or MR according to the theoretical foundation of these methods.

Provided that the investigated compounds can be described as a rigid backbone plus substituents at various sites (Cammarata and Menon, 1976), the best way to translate the structural variation to numbers is to use "substituent scales" such as pi of Hansch and Leo (1979), sigma of Hammett (1970) or Taft (1956), E_s of Taft (1956), etc. These scales are derived from chemical model reactions and thereby have the right properties to constitute x-variables in PARC and MR. Moreover, with a sufficient range of model reactions, one can hope to catch all possible "effects" of substituents.

These empirical parameters can, naturally, be supplemented with "theoretically" derived descriptors such as the steric constants of Verloop *et al.* (1976), and quantum mechanical charges and electro-negativities (e.g. Gasteiger and Jochum, 1978).

To describe interactions between substituent sites, squared terms and cross-terms can be introduced as additional descriptors. In the end, this may lead to a large number of descriptors, but with proper data analysis this is no problem.

The phenethylamines in the example (see Fig. 2) have a semi-rigid backbone plus four substituent sites. The substituent in the phenyl group was described by f of Rekker (1977), sigma and L and B_4 of Verloop *et al.* (1976). R_1 was described by its f-value and R_2 by f, sigma and E_s plus the calculated pK_a of the amino-group. Three additional descriptors for the meta position in the phenyl group were found irrelevant in an earlier investigation (Dunn *et al.*, 1978) and not included. No cross-terms or squares were used. Hence, in total nine variables are used to describe the structural variation between the 37 compounds.

Flexible molecules

In larger aliphatic compounds, peptides, etc., with flexible conformations, it is often very difficult to separate the molecular structure
into "backbone" and "substituents" unless one has direct information
(e.g. X-ray) about the conformation when bound to the receptor or the
"active site". One must then try other ways to quantify the structural
variation. Descriptors derived from molecular mechanics and "exclusion
volumes" as discussed by Garland Marshall at this meeting (see Chapter
3) may be an interesting appraoch.

The successful applications of PARC to QSAR for flexible compounds are still rare, in our view mainly because of lack of knowledge
of how to translate the variation in their chemical structure to relevant
variables.

Geometrical Representation of PARC

Once we have managed to transform our problem into finding relations
in and between two matrices X and Y, the data analysis can start. It is
convenient to regard PARC as the spatial analysis of point configur-
ations in a multidimensional space. Thus, if we let each of the p x-
variables define one orthogonal coordinate axis, we get a p-dimensional
space in which the X-data of one compound constitute a single point.
We shall call this space "M-space" (measurement space, multivariate
space), "X-space" (representing X) or "p-space" (p-dimensional)
depending on the context. Analogously, the q y-values of one compound
are represented as a point in the q-dimensional Y-space or "E-space"
(effect-space) or "q-space".

In the present example, the X-space has eight dimensions and Y-space
two or three for the antagonists and agonists, respectively. Spaces with
more than three dimensions are difficult to visualize. Mathematically,
however, they are defined and can be manipulated by a computer.
Points, lines, planes, angles and distances have the same meaning in
p-space when $p > 3$ as with $p = 2$ or 3. We therefore use 3-spaces as
illustrations and remember that the same things go on in higher dimensional spaces, only "much more".

If we have two classes of compounds as in the example, and if the
X-data contain any information about the class difference, the point
swarms of the two classes will in some way be situated in different
regions in M-space as illustrated in Fig. 3. Though one can imagine
strange class shapes in M-space with intricately entangled classes, simple
theoretical arguments indicate that this rarely or never happens in
practice. As long as the compounds in a class are similar, the class will
have a simple shape and can be well approximated by a bilinear model

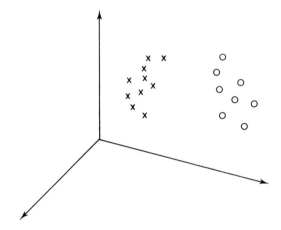

FIG. 3   The data vector of one object (the x part) is represented by a point in the p-dimensional space spanned by the p x-variables. Though spaces with $p > 3$ are difficult to visualize, three-dimensional spaces can be used as illustrations. Points, lines, planes, angles and distances have the same properties in spaces with many dimensions as in those with two or three.

such as the principal components (PC) and partial least squares (PLS) models used in SIMCA (Wold, 1976).

Common Methods of PARC

All methods commonly used in medical chemistry (i.e. non-linguistic methods) can be seen as in one way or another describing either (i) the separation or (ii) the location of the class "point swarms" in M-space.

Figures 4–7 show geometrical representations of the most common PARC methods linear discriminant analysis (LDA) and the closely related linear learning machine (LLM), K^{th} nearest neighbour method (KNN), Bayesean methods (BM) and SIMCA (soft independent modelling of class analogy).

Of these methods, LDA and LLM have the disadvantage of being unable to operate with many x-variables; the condition is that $p < n/3$ for these methods. They are therefore very sensitive to the presence of strong subgroups in classes since this decreases the "practical n" (Wold and Dunn, 1983). These drawbacks make these methods of limited utility in drug design.

The KNN method is stable and gives good results as long as each class has about the same size of its training set and as long as the x-variables are not scaled to enhance the class separation (Fisher or variance–weight scaling). Autoscaling the data to unit variance for each variable over the training set (Kowalski and Bender, 1972) is recommended, in order

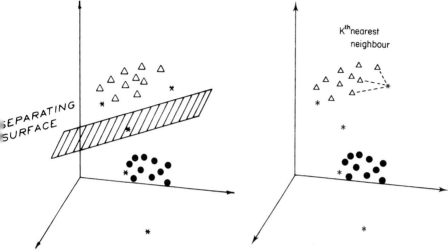

FIG. 4 With linear discriminant analysis (LDA) and the linear learning machine (LLM), the classes are separated in M-space by a p-1 dimensional plane.

FIG. 5 The Kth nearest neighbour (KNN) method classifies test set objects (asterisk) according to the class of the Kth nearest neighbour (usually K = 1 or 3).

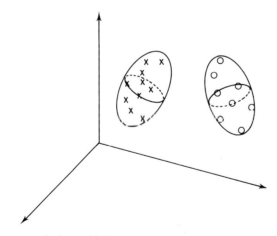

FIG. 6 In Bayesean methods, empirical distributions are calculated for each model. In a simple case, a class is described by the mean and standard deviation of each variable (2 p parameters), but in realistic models, the covariances between the variables must also be included (2 p + p(p − 1)/2 param.s).

not to overestimate the class separation. With well represented training sets, KNN can operate also on PARC level 3. The predicted activity for test set compounds is then a weighted average of the activities of its Kth nearest neighbour.

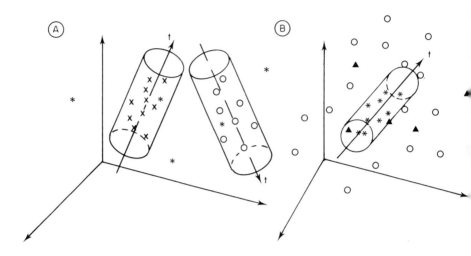

FIG. 7a   Same as figure 3, but with one-dimensional PC models (lines) fitted separately to each class. Tolerance regions have been constructed around each class (cylinders) on the basis of the scatter of the training set points around the models. Test set points (asterisks) are classified according to their positions inside or outside class cylinders.

FIG. 7b   The asymmetric (embedded) data structure, where one class is "tightly" structured and can be described by a PC model (here one-dimensional as an example), while the second class is not a "proper" class with similar objects, and thus cannot be modelled. SIMCA classification is still accomplished by judging the position of an object as inside or outside the confidence region of the "tight" class. This type of classification is closely related to control theory and acceptance regions.

Bayesean methods have good properties when the data set is large, i.e. has many objects. Then distribution models for each class can be estimated and new compounds assigned to the class to the distribution of which they fit best. Since the number of compounds in QSAR and drug design is rarely large, these methods are seldom used in this field.

SIMCA

On PARC levels 1 and 2, when only X-data are given and the purpose is to find rules for the classification of "objects" on the basis of these data, SIMCA operates by fitting disjoint principal components (PC) models separately to each class "point swarm". This corresponds to the decomposition of the scaled class matrix X_g (class g) into a class average vector, $\underline{x}$, loading vectors $\underline{b}$, and score vectors $\underline{t}$. Thus the place of each compound inside the class is described by coordinates t (see Fig. 7).

Since only the first few principal components of X_g are used to model a class, this analysis can be done even when the number of x-variables, p, is large. In fact, the values of t_a become more stable the larger p is, since they have the properties of weighted averages of all the x-variables.

The PC analysis and the PLS analysis (see below) work also with moderate amounts of missing data (say, less than 30%) provided that these are not missing in "systematic patterns" that differ between the classes.

Scaling of the data   PC modelling is a variance maximizing method, the results of which depend on the scaling of the data. When information is available about the relative importance of the variables, they should be weighted to have an original variance proportional to this importance. In the usual case, when such information is lacking, the recommended scaling is to normalize each variable to unit variance within each class, i.e. disjoint class scaling (Wold *et al.*, 1983).

Minimum size of the training set   To estimate PC models of any stability for the classes in the training set, at least five compounds are needed in each class and ten or more are preferable.

Level 3   In a level 3 problem, one may then investigate whether, for instance, highly active compounds are situated in a "corner" of the class or in some other subregion. This is done simply by using the compound coordinates in the class, t_a (one for each model dimension a) as independent variables in a standard multiple regression (MR) with the activity y as dependent variable. Curved relationships are handled by including the squares of the coordinates t in the MR. Cross-terms are unnecessary since the different coordinate vectors t_a are orthogonal to each other.

Level 4   On level 4, with several y-variables, disjoint models for each class are constructed also in Y-space. The place of a compound in a class is there described by coordinates u_a, which are summaries of all the activities y_q. These u-values can then be used as dependent variables in the MR model, which thus gives a relation between the X and Y parts of the class data (Fig. 8).

In the analysis of PARC 4 problems with more than, say, five or six y-variables, the variation in Y can be separated into three parts. First, a separate PC analysis of the Y-matrix of a class separates the variation in Y into systematic part, "signal" and "noise". Then in the PLS analysis (see below) relating Y to X, one gets a measure of how much of the variation in Y is "explained" by X. The difference between the two measures, the lack of information in X about Y, provides useful indications on where to improve the models.

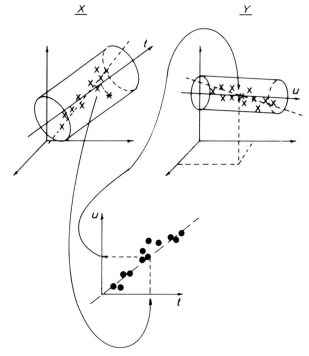

FIG. 8   In PARC levels 3 and 4, relations between the X-block and the Y-block of variables are constructed separately for each separate class. With the PLS method, this can be illustrated as relations between constructs in one space for the x-data and one space for the y-data. On level 3 with only one y-variable, the latter space is one-dimensional.

In the training phase, models similar to PC models are constructed that approximate the X and Y data of a class. These models are tilted slightly to improve the correlation between the classes in terms of the correlation between the projection t and the projection u (lower part of the figure). Tolerance intervals (cylinders) are constructed just as in SIMCA level 2 (Fig. 7).

In the "test phase", the prediction phase, a new object (asterisk) is classified as similar to the class or not according to its position inside or outside the class tolerance interval in X-space. The position of the object point along the x-part of the model, i.e. the coordinate t, is introduced in the u-t-plot (lower part of the picture) which gives a predicted u-value for the object. This is taken into the model in Y-space to give predicted values of each of the y-variables.

Phase 2, classification and prediction of Y   In the second phase of the analysis, test set compounds are classified on the basis of their structure descriptors x. If the test set compound in M-space falls inside a class "cylinder", it is assigned to this class. This also gives the projection down on the class PC model (line or plane), i.e. the t-values of the compound. On level 3 or 4, these then are inserted into the MR model to give predicted values for the biological activities of the compound, y.

If the data X are not sufficient to separate the classes, the class models and their tolerance cylinders will overlap in some regions. A new compound might then be classified as belonging to two or several classes and on level 3 and 4 one gets several sets of predicted y-values. The only way to improve this situation is to improve the description of the structures of the compounds, i.e. to have additional and more relevant X-data.

It may also happen that a compound is far outside all class "cylinders". It is then an "outlier" of a new type and no predictions about its activities can be made.

PLS A numerically and statistically more efficient way to analyse the level 3 and 4 problem is to use the PLS method of H. Wold (1982). This combines the principal components analysis and the multiple regression in one single step. Thereby the information in the data is used more efficiently which gives a better predictive model of Y. Geometrically, the PLS method has the same representation as that of principal components, with the "inner PLS relation" being a linear model between t and u (or y on level 3) as shown in Fig. 8.

The Example

We have p = 9 x-variables describing the structural variation among the substituted phenethylamines and q = 2 or 3 y-variables related to their beta-adrenergic activity. Hence, this is a PARC 4 problem. Using the PLS method with cross-validation, we find that three-dimensional models adequately describe the X-data of both the antagonist and agonist classes. These models reclassify most of the compounds correctly as shown in the standard decision diagram (SDD), in Fig. 9. The models also show a good predictive relation between the X and Y-blocks of each class (Fig. 10 and 11). The model parameters are given in Table 2.

Hence we conclude that the nine structure descriptors x_k are useful to classify compounds of this type as antagonists or agonists and also can predict the level of the measured beta-adrenergic activities of the compounds. This does not mean that the set of descriptors is the best one. On the contrary, the inclusion of other relevant descriptors will probably improve both the classification and the prediction of Y. But the present set is sufficient for the purpose of the investigation; to show that there are systematic structural differences between the two classes and that the structural variation within each class is related to the level of biological activity.

The structure of new compounds, like the five test set compounds, can now be translated to the values of 9 descriptors. These define points in 9-space which are inside one or the other class cylinders, or inside both or neither. Thereby they are classified as antagonist, agonist,

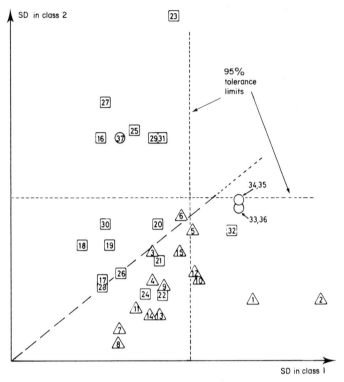

FIG. 9   Distance (residual standard deviation) to class model 1 plotted against distance to class model 2 for the compounds (class 1, class 2, test set). Dashed line indicates the border between the two classes. Nos 22, 24 and 32 are clearly incorrectly classified.

TABLE 2a

Loadings and modelling power for variables in class 1. Data class-scaled

Variable	Beta-1	Beta-2	Beta-3	Mpow
y-1	0.75	0.64	0 75	0.94
y-2	0.66	0.77	0.66	0.86
x-1	0.08	−0.34	0.13	0.20
x-2	−0.20	0.64	0.13	0.88
x-3	0.29	−0.25	0.03	0.53
x-4	0.48	0.24	−0.05	0.97
x-5	−0.43	0.06	0.02	0.78
x-6	−0.46	−0.07	0.11	0.89
x-7	−0.21	−0.34	0.62	0.81
x-8	0.36	−0.34	0.07	0.78
x-9	0.26	−0.32	0.75	0.97

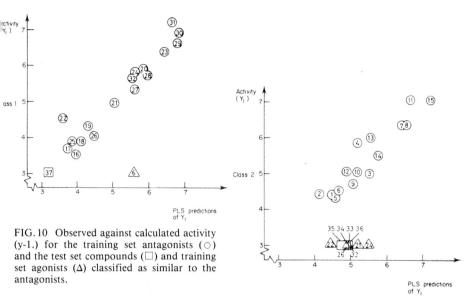

FIG. 10 Observed against calculated activity (y-1.) for the training set antagonists (○) and the test set compounds (□) and training set agonists (Δ) classified as similar to the antagonists.

FIG. 11 Observed against calculated activity (y-1.) for the training set agonists (○)and the test set compounds (□) and training set antagonists (Δ) classified as similar to the agonists.

possibly both or neither. If a point is inside a class cylinder, predicted values for the y-variables are obtained as indicated in Fig. 8.

The results of this analysis of the test set are included in Figs 9 to 11. Compound 37 is classified as a very weak but clear antagonist, while nos 33–36 are correctly classified as borderline cases with very weak or absent activity.

TABLE 2b

Loadings and modelling power for variables in class 2. Data class-scaled

Variable	Beta-1	Beta-2	Beta-3	Mpow
y-1	0.73	0.49	0.00	0.93
y-2	0.66	0.57	−0.28	0.92
y-3	−0.19	0.66	0.96	0.83
x-1	0.16	−0.94	0.12	0.99
x-2	−0.29	0.03	0.85	0.97
x-3	−0.40	−0.12	0.08	0.62
x-4	0.46	−0.21	0.32	0.87
x-5	−0.50	0.22	−0.22	0.94
x-6	−0.52	0.02	−0.33	0.98

Summary of SIMCA/PLS

In the SIMCA method, empirical models are constructed for each proper class. The modelling power listed in Table 2 gives information about the systematic behaviour of the x-variables inside each class. The model parameters are also useful for the interpretation of the class structure. Training set objects far from their "own" class model are outliers, anomalous compounds or compounds having erroneous initial class assignment or incorrectly entered data.

The models are used to classify test set objects and, on levels 3 and 4, to predict values of dependent variables y.

The development of a PC model demands at least five and preferably ten or more compounds in a class.

Since each class is analysed independently of the others, the method works as well with few as with many classes.

The method works with any number of x- and y-variables, in contrast to regression methods and linear discriminant analysis and the linear learning machine. The results of both classification and prediction become more stable the larger the number of relevant x- and y-variables.

Moderate amounts of "missing data" can be handled efficiently by the method. If the missing data are not distributed randomly and if the missing data distribution differs between the classes, one must however, be careful that one does not get artifacts caused by the missing data "patterns".

With many y-variables (more than five or six), the variation in Y can be separated into systematic part "explained" by X, systematic part not "explained" by X and noise.

The method works also in the case of asymmetric (embedded) data structures (Dunn and Wold, 1980b). This case is rather common in QSAR applications where one well defined class of active compounds is contrasted to a diffuse class containing all other possibilities, i.e. inactive compounds. In this case, the data often have the structure in M-space such that the first class defines a tight cluster which can be modelled by a simple PC model, while the second class cannot be modelled. With SIMCA a classification is still obtained; objects inside the tolerance "cylinder" of the first class are assigned to this class while objects outside the cylinder are assigned to the "all others" class, i.e. inactive. Since the "classes" are not linearly separable, LDA and LLM are not applicable and will give poor results.

Conclusion

The reason for using PARC in QSAR is that in many problems it is difficult to describe the variation in structure between investigated compounds with one or a few descriptors. When a larger number of descriptors, possibly relevant, possibly irrelevant, are to be analysed in relation to possibly multivariate activity data, and when the compounds are divided into different structural and/or pharmacological classes, the traditional regression methods are less useful and PARC is the only possible approach.

The analysis is done in several steps, each of which involves many possibilities for going wrong. However, the experience of PARC applied in chemistry and QSAR makes it possible to give guidelines which, if followed, increase the probability substantially that the results of the analysis are reliable.

It should be noted that the adoption of these guidelines increases the power of the methodology in that if a problem is badly specified or if the structure data X are irrelevant, the results of the analysis tend to be negative. From the scientific point of view this is desirable, but it leads to fewer publications than if one uses a methodology which always gives apparently good correlations.

1) Problem specification and formulation. Think carefully about your compounds and their drug activity (and side-effects) you wish to model. Divide the compounds into classes corresponding to different structural types and different pharmacological mechanisms. Regard this as a tentative division, which might have to be changed with reassignments and further splits later on in the investigation.

2) Select relevant variables to describe the structural variation among the compounds. Try to use variables derived from real measurements (e.g. pi, sigma, E_s) and theoretical variables you understand (like charges, polarizabilities, electro-negativities). If you have access to data describing the influence of your "substituents" on biological activities, e.g. earlier investigated drug series, this is ideal. Do not use fragment occurrences as one−zero variables. Avoid other one−zero variables.

Do not use a scheme of variable selection because the statistical risks for spurious correlations are then substantial (Topliss and Edwards, 1979). Instead, use all your variables in the analysis.

3) Select representative compounds for the training set. Do not vary one substituent site at a time. Try to get combinations of acceptors, halogens, alkyls, donors and hydrogen spread over all sites of substitution plus a variation in total lipophilicity.

4) Make relevant (and preferably several different) biological activity measurements on your compounds. Repeat the measurements for a few compounds after a while without telling the pharmacologists. This gives you a good idea of the precision of the data.

5) Analyse your data with an appropriate method. If you have more than ten x-variables, do not use LDA or LLM or multiple regression. Take out projection plots (principal components, factor score plots, eigenvector plots) of your X- and Y-space. Look for groupings inside your classes, outliers, strange patterns. Check the input data for outliers. Look for indications for an asymmetric data structure; if positive then use KNN or SIMCA/PLS.

Do not be disappointed by negative results. They are useful because they force you to think. QSAR and drug design is difficult; presently the most challenging area of chemistry and pharmacology.

6) Validate your results by keeping a quarter of your data set, selected at random, out of the first phase of the analysis. Then reclassify these compounds and predict their y-values with the models derived from the remaining three quarters of the data. If the results are no better than guessing, think. Then return to step one.

7) Try to interpret your results. Twist the problem formulation and the data set and the way of analysis and have another go, with new plots, etc.

8) Verify interesting results by making compounds and testing them. This is the only really reliable way to check the validity of your data analysis and your models. If, too often, you get much worse results than predicted, think about your choice of classes, compounds, descriptors and data analytic method.

Acknowledgements

Grants from the Swedish Natural Science Research Council (NFR), the Swedish Council for Planning and Coordination of Research (FRN) and the National Swedish Board for Technical Development (STU) are gratefully acknowledged.

References

Albano, C., Dunn, W.J. III, Edlund, U. *et al.* (1978). *Anal. Chim. Acta Comput. Tech. Optim.* **103**, 429–443.
Box, G.E.P., Hunter, W.G. and Hunter, J.S. (1978). "Statistics for Experimenters". Wiley, New York.

Cammarata, A. and Menon, G.K. (1976). *J. Med. Chem.* **19**, 739–748.
Dunn, W.J., Wold, S. and Martin, Y.C. (1978). *J. Med. Chem.* **21**, 922–930.
Dunn, W.J. and Wold, S. (1980a). *Bioorg. Chem.* **9**, 505–523.
Dunn, W.J. and Wold, S. (1980b). *J. Med. Chem.* **23**, 595–599.
Gasteiger, J. and Jochum, C. (1978). *Top. Curr. Chem.* **74**, 93.
Hammett, L.P. (1970). "Physical Organic Chemistry", 2nd edn, McGraw-Hill, New York.
Hansch, C. and Leo, A.J. (1979). "Substituent Constants for Correlation Analysis in Chemistry and Biology". Wiley, New York.
Kowalski, B.R. and Bender, C.F. (1972). *J. Amer. Chem. Soc.* **94**, 5632–5639.
Mukherjee, C., Caron, M.G., Mullikin, D. and Lefkowitz, R.J. (1976). *Mol. Pharmacology* **12**, 16.
Redl, G., Cramer, R.D. III and Berkhoff, C.E. (1974). *Chem. Soc. Rev.* **3**, 273.
Rekker, R.F. (1977). "The Hydrophobic Fragment Constant". Elsevier, Amsterdam.
Taft, R.W. (1956). *In* "Steric Effects in Organic Chemistry" (M.S. Newman, ed.), Ch. 13. Wiley, New York.
Topliss, J.G. and Edwards, R.P. (1979). *J. Med. Chem.* **22**, 1238–1244.
Verloop, A., Hoogenstraaten, W. and Tipker, J. (1976). *In* "Drug Design", Vol. 7 (E.J. Ariens, ed.), pp. 101–146. Academic Press, New York.
Wold, H. (1982). *In* "Systems Under Indirect Observation" (K.G. Joreskog and H. Wold, eds), pp. 1–54. North-Holland, Amsterdam.
Wold, S. (1976). *Pattern Recognition* **8**, 127–139.
Wold, S., Dunn, W.J. III, and Hellberg, S. (1982). Survey of Applications of Pattern Recognition to Structure-Activity Problems. Tech. Rep. R.G. Chemometrics, Umeå University.
Wold, S. and Dunn, W.J. III (1983). Multivariate Quantitative Structure–Activity Relationships (QSAR): conditions for their applicability. *J. Chem. Inf. Comput. Sci.* **23**, 6–13.
Wold, S., Albano, C., Dunn III, W.J. and others.(1983). *In* Pattern Recognition: Finding and Using Regularities in Multivariate Data. Proc. IUFOST Conf. Food Research and Data Analysis (H. Martens, ed.), pp. 147–188. Elsevier, Amsterdam.

Discussion

Chairman: Professor Tomlinson

Professor Andrews

Dr Wold suggested that we should be measuring as many different biological activities as possible, and that further, we should be looking at as many different chemical variables too in the use of pattern recognition. What about the situation when each of the individual drug molecules at which we are looking can also adopt a number of different conformations, for example? Can that problem be handled with pattern recognition?

Dr Wold

I do not think this is a problem of pattern recognition, but a problem of how to describe the structure of flexible molecules quantitatively. Once that can be done, it can be fed into pattern recognition. However, I do not think that at present we are very good at that. I think that the approach of Professor Marshall may be a basis to do that, but have not done much with it yet.

The only promising approach that I can see is to try to get some idea about the possible variation of flexible molecules, and then to describe that quantitatively and translate it to a number of variables, using it in pattern recognition. That has not yet been done, however.

Professor Andrews
The problem with that is that while Professor Marshall's approach offers a series of alternative molecules and the space that they are likely to occupy, it does not really take into account the relative likelihood of the existence of different conformations.

Dr Wold
But that can also be done in his approach, I think, if it is developed — that is for debate between the two of you.

Dr Choplin
In answer to Professor Andrew's question, there may be a possible method of describing the molecule with its conformation. It is the relatively new technique of autocorrelation vectors, dealing with three-dimensional representation of the molecule, as described recently by Dr Moreau from Roussel. This could be a technique enabling the description of the entire molecule without any bias — it is an unbiased representation — and it can take into account the complete three-dimensional representation of the molecule.

Dr Wold
But the problem with this work is that his evaluation is based on wrong statistics. He has not shown, therefore, that it is a valid approach.

Dr Choplin
I do not know whether I agree with Dr Wold, but the problem of representation could be solved by this means. He uses learning-machine techniques, but I think that using this type of representation with simple factor analysis would give better results.

Dr Wold
I agree with Dr Choplin — this should be tried.

Professor Marshall
It seems to me that one of the messages which is slowly but surely beginning to penetrate the fog is the following. I was raised on the prejudice that we want to get as few variables as possible, so that something like this Fourier transform of a molecule description ends up with one, or a small set of quantities, of something which is really an elaborate set of properties. But, from what I hear from Dr Wold, if we can calculate that elaborate set, we can put them in and let the statistics throw out the things that do not matter. Thus, in many ways, the more properties, the more variables, the more complex description that we have of our system, probably the better off we shall be.

Dr Wold

On one condition − it can be shown that the information content (if the analysis is done properly) increases as the square root of the number of relevant variables. As long as the structure is described in a more relevant and better way by adding more descriptors, that will be related in a better way to the present activity problem. Things will then work better. There is thus no basic need to look at only a few variables, but this does not mean that we can introduce the whole universe of descriptors in each problem. That is because if a majority of the descriptors have nothing to do with the particular problem, they introduce noise in which the relevant variables drown. We still have to *think* − that is the problem with which we always end up.

7 Pharmacological Receptors and Drug Design

B.P. ROQUES

*Département de Chimie Organique, U.E.R. des
Sciences Pharmaceutiques et Biologiques,
Université René Descartes, 4 Avenue de
l'Observatoire, 75270 Paris Cedex 06, France*

Introduction

Molecular pharmacology can be considered as a new discipline, the aim
of which is to correct or to restore a deficient physiological mechanism.
The development of our knowledge of the molecular structures of
various pharmacological targets such as nucleic acids, receptors of the
central nervous system or neuropeptidases allows a rational design of
probes to investigate their mechanism of action and possibly the synthesis of new active drugs. For such a purpose physicochemical methods
such as NMR spectroscopy, fluorescence techniques and binding experiments have been of great value. This molecular approach, systematically used in our laboratory during the last ten years will be illustrated
by two examples: the synthesis of DNA bis-intercalators as new antitumour drugs and the differentiation of μ and δ opiate receptors as a
novel aid in the search for analgesic and psychoactive agents.

DNA Bis-Intercalators: a New Class of Antitumour Agents*

It is more and more probable that tumoral genes belong to the regular
genomic content of all cells. The malignant cell-transformation would

---

* This work was performed in close collaboration with Professor J.B. Le Pecq and his co-workers
(Laboratoire de Pharmacologie Moléculaire du C.N.R.S., Villejuif).

DRUG DESIGN: FACT OR FANTASY
ISBN 0.12.388180.3

occur through successive induction (by chemical or viral agents) and promotion mechanisms leading to the final expression of cancer gene(s). Chemical modifications of the DNA are usually deleted by several repair enzymes but such enzymatic processes seem to be partially at fault within the tumour cells (Dulbecco, 1982).

Moreover, genomic activation occurs through structural changes of chromatin, i.e. a relaxation process, increasing the accessibility of exogenous toxic agents to the DNA base pairs. Therefore these recent results could provide a molecular explanation for both the carcino-genesis and the higher sensitivity of the transformed cells to drugs which affect division.

Along these lines, it is of considerable interest to observe that several highly potent and clinically used anticancer agents such as actinomycin, daunorubicin, doxorubicin and ellipticine interact with nucleic acids according to the intercalation concept (Lerman, 1961).

However, affinity constants of intercalating agents are in the region of $10^5 M^{-1}$, far from the affinity constants of proteins such as re-pressors or RNA polymerase which bind to DNA with $K_A = 10^{10}$ to $10^{12} M^{-1}$. Obviously these molecules can easily displace classical inter-calating agents. In order to possibly enhance the antitumour properties of this kind of drug, we have sought molecules able to compete with these proteins for DNA. Taking into account that repressor proteins and RNA polymerase are oligomeric, we have developed dimeric mole-cules made up of two intercalating moieties linked by aminoalkyl chains of various lengths. Theoretical approach, synthesis and conformational properties of DNA bis-intercalators as well as binding properties and antitumour activity were successively investigated. Some results of these studies will be reported here.

Theoretical binding affinity of dimeric effectors with biological targets

Following a simple thermodynamic concept the reversible bimolecular association between a monomeric effector K_{mon} and a complementary structure is related to the maximum free energy change ΔG_{mon} by the relation:

$$\Delta G_{mon} = RT \, Ln \, K_{mon}.$$

Appropriate dimerization of this monomeric effector leads to identical sub-units able to interact simultaneously with two complementary sym-metrical targets. The free energy change of such a bis-interaction corresponds theoretically to:

$$\Delta G_{dim} = 2\Delta G_{mon} - RT \, Ln \, X,$$

where X = molar concentration of water in solution.

Since the term $RT \, Ln \, X$, which corresponds to the entropy of mixing, is weak the theoretical maximum binding affinity of a dimeric molecule will be given by:

$$RT \, Ln \, K_{dim} = 2 \, RT \, Ln \, K_{mon} , \qquad (K_{dim})_{max} \sim K^2_{mon}$$

Obviously, this theoretical value will always be decreased by the loss of free energy related to conformational restriction in the degree of freedom accounted for by dimerization.

Design and Conformational Properties of DNA Bis-Intercalators

In order to investigate the topological concept of DNA bis-intercalation, we first prepared dimers made up of acridine or ethidium rings linked by various aminoalkyl chains (Fig. 1).

Although devoid of significant antitumour properties, these heterocycles were selected as intercalating moieties owing to the well-known enhancement of their native fluorescence upon DNA intercalation (Markovits *et al.*, 1979).

Based on this property, a new kinetic method allowing the determination of very high affinity constants was developed and used to verify that dimerization led indeed to molecules able to bind to DNA with K_A in the range of $10^8 M^{-1}$ to $10^{11} M^{-1}$ (Barbet *et al.*, 1975; Le Pecq *et al.*, 1975; Roques *et al.*, 1976a; Gaugain *et al.*, 1978b; Capelle *et al.*, 1979; Markovits *et al.*, 1981a)

Starting from these promising results, we replaced the preceding heterocycles with larger aromatic rings such as "ellipticine", which displays by itself strong antitumour properties (Juret *et al.*, 1982), and the four isomeric 7H-pyridocarbazoles (Pelaprat *et al.*, 1980a).

All the intercalating moieties used to synthesize bis-intercalators are highly hydrophobic and therefore self-associate in aqueous solution with association constants between $100 \, M^{-1}$ to $5000 \, M^{-1}$ (Delbarre *et al.*, 1977; Laugâa *et al.*, 1981). In the case of dimeric compounds the aromatic rings linked by flexible chains stack one above another leading to intramolecularly stacked forms strongly stabilized at physiological pH (Barbet *et al.*, 1976; Roques *et al.*, 1976b; Delbarre *et al.*, 1981). This feature is very unfavourable for DNA bis-intercalation since this process obviously requires the opening of the folded form. Moreover, in the stacked conformation the proximity between the charged intercalating rings decreases the pKa of the nitrogen of the linking chain and therefore

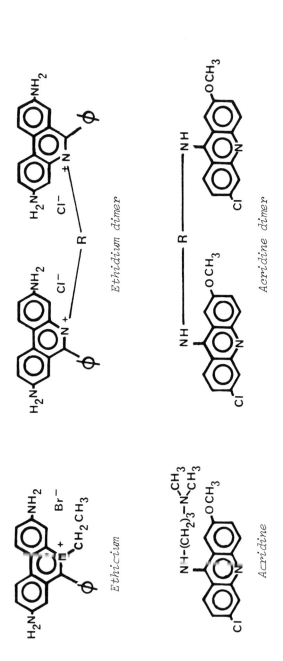

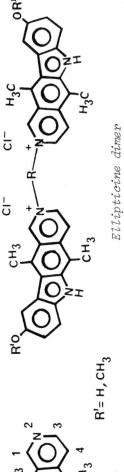

Ethidium

Ethidium dimer

Acridine

Acridine dimer

Ellipticine
(6H-pyridocarbazole)

Ellipticine dimer

R'= H, CH₃

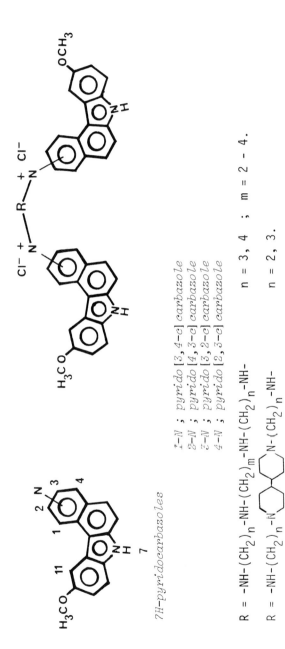

7H-pyridocarbazoles

1-N ; pyrido [3,4-c] carbazole
2-N ; pyrido [4,3-c] carbazole
3-N ; pyrido [3,2-c] carbazole
4-N ; pyrido [2,3-c] carbazole

R = -NH-(CH₂)ₙ-NH-(CH₂)ₘ-NH-(CH₂)ₙ-NH-   n = 3, 4 ; m = 2 - 4.

R = -NH-(CH₂)ₙ-N⟨ ⟩N-(CH₂)ₙ-NH-   n = 2, 3.

FIG. 1   Structure of different DNA intercalating agents under their monomeric or dimeric forms and of some alkylamino chains used as spacers.

removes the electrostatic interaction of the spacer with the negatively charged DNA ribose–phosphate backbone.

In order to overcome all these unfavourable conformational features, we synthesized a new series of bis-intercalators bearing rigid linking chains. When quaternized by the ethyl bis-piperidine spacer, the distance between the pyridocarbazolium rings corresponds exactly to that required for bis-intercalation by the energetically favoured "excluded site model" (Bauer *et al.*, 1970), Fig. 2 (a).

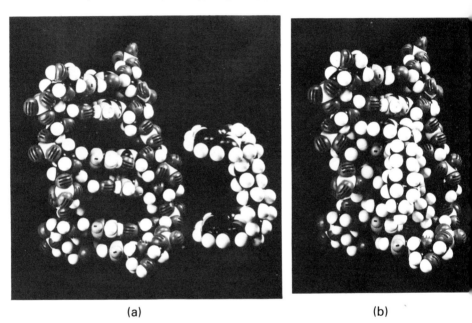

(a)   (b)

FIG. 2   CPK space filling molecular models of DNA.
(a) DNA with two intercalating-sites according to the excluded-site model (left) and preferential conformation of the rigid dimer exhibiting antitumour property: 1,1′-bis-[2-(10-methoxy, 7H-pyrido[4,3-c]carbazolium) ethyl]-4,4′-bipiperidine (right).
(b) DNA bis-intercalating complex of the rigid dimer.

Moreover, as expected this kind of rigid chain inhibits intramolecular stacking interactions as clearly shown by the similarity between the spectra of the monomeric acridine and the derived rigid dimer, whereas the aromatic protons of the flexible dimer are shifted strongly upfield by the shielding current of the superimposed ring (Fig. 3). Finally, it must be underlined that, in the rigid dimer, distinct signals are observed for axial and equatorial protons of the bis-piperidine moiety, even at pH 7.4 when the chain is uncharged. This demonstrates the rigidity of the bis-(ethylpiperidinyl) bridge under physiological conditions. In contrast, in the corresponding monomer the chemical shifts are averaged

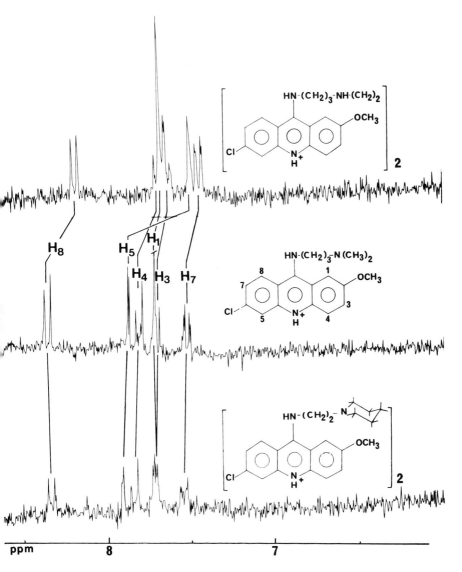

FIG. 3 Aromatic part of ^{1}H NMR spectra of acridine monomer (middle), flexible (top) and rigid (bottom) dimers performed at 270 MHz in D_2O (10^{-4}M, pH 5.6; temp, 21°C; TMS as internal reference). Redrawn from Deibarre *et al.*, 1981.

by the rapid equilibrium between different conformations of the piperidine ring (Delbarre *et al.*, 1981).

Biological Properties of DNA Bis-Intercalators

The intercalation of a given compound between stacked base pairs of DNA induces both a lengthening and an unwinding of the double helix. These changes can be evidenced through viscosimetric experiments. Thus, taking into account that the length of short pieces of sonicated calf thymus DNA increases by 3.4 Å upon intercalation, the variations of log η/η_o versus log $(1 + 2r)$ leads to slopes between 2.3 and 3 for monointercalation and higher than 4 in the case of bis-intercalation. In the preceding equation, η and η_o are respectively the intrinsic viscosity of sonicated DNA in the presence and in the absence of a given compound and r is the ratio of the molar concentration of the bound molecule to the molar concentration of DNA nucleotides (Saucier *et al.*, 1971; Butour *et al.*, 1978).

Likewise, the bis-intercalating character of a compound can be verified by measuring the unwinding of supercoiled PM-2 DNA (Waring, 1970, Revet *et al.*, 1971), at pH 5. In this assay, the value of the unwinding angle induced by a bis-intercalator must be almost twice that caused by the corresponding monomer (Le Pecq *et al.*, 1975).

Some comparative results corresponding to the 7H-pyridocarbazole series are reported in Table 1. They clearly indicate that dimers **3** and **4**

TABLE 1

DNA binding affinity and intercalation parameters of some 7H-pyrido[4,3-c]carbazoles

Compounds	R	n	K_{ap} $(M^{-1})^a$	Slope $(1+2r)^b$	Unwinding angle[c]
1	H	1	5.2×10^5	2.5	14.5°
2	CH_3	1	1.8×10^6	2.8	ND
3	H	2	5.0×10^8	4.4	21.6°
4	CH_3	2	3.0×10^8	5.6	ND

[a] Binding constants were measured by displacement of ethidium or ethidium dimer bound to calf thymus DNA. [b] Slope of the reduced viscosimetry of sonicated DNA as a function of the number of molecules of compound bound per nucleotide. [c] Unwinding of covalently closed DNA from PM$_2$ phage. Details of these experiments were reported in Pelaprat *et al.*, 1980a; Pelaprat *et al.*, 1980b.

behave as DNA bis-intercalators. Similar results were obtained in the case of acridine dimers (Le Pecq *et al.*, 1975; Capelle *et al.*, 1979) whereas ethidium dimer only mono-intercalates (Gaugain *et al.*, 1978b; Markovits *et al.*, 1979). These compounds were used to determine the DNA affinity constants, K_A, of bis-intercalating dimers. Because of the very high K_A's of such compounds ($> 10^8 M^{-1}$), classical binding isotherms by fluorescence techniques cannot be used since the sensitivity of these methods is insufficient to measure the difference between free and bound molecules at concentrations below $10^{-7} M$.

Therefore a new kinetic method was employed to estimate the K_As of bis-intercalators using one acridine dimer as model (Capelle *et al.*, 1979). Stopped-flow experiments led to the determination of on-rate constants from the time-dependent increase in fluorescence of the dimer upon its binding to poly (dA−dT). Association constants ($\sim 3 \times 10^7 M^{-1} s^{-1}$) were found for monomeric and dimeric acridines. Utilizing the fluorescence quenching of acridine bound to a G−C base pair, off-rate constants were estimated from exchange experiments between poly(dA−dT) and G−C rich *Micrococcus luteus* DNA. The dissociation constant was found very small ($k_{off} \sim 1.5 \times 10^{-3} s^{-1}$) for the acridine dimer. Therefore its estimated DNA binding $K_A = k_{on}/k_{off} \sim 2 \times 10^{10} M^{-1}$ is more than 50 000 times larger than the corresponding constant of the acridine monomer, in good accordance with the theoretical concept (Le Pecq *et al.*, 1975).

Obviously kinetic experiments cannot be performed with non-fluorescent compounds such as the 7H-pyridocarbazole dimers, whose DNA and RNA affinity constants were determined by competition with the highly fluorescent ethidium dimer (Gaugain *et al.*, 1978b; Markovits *et al.*, 1981b; Reinhardt *et al.*, 1982). The smaller DNA affinity of compounds 3 and 4, $K_A \sim 10^8 M^{-1}$ (Table 1) as compared to acridine dimers could be due to the larger size of the pyridocarbazole rings leading to an unfavourable entropic factor in the DNA bis-intercalation process. Nevertheless the DNA binding affinities of these bis-intercalators are about 1000 times higher than those of the corresponding monomers (Pelaprat *et al.*, 1980b).

Geometries of the DNA Intercalating Complexes of Various Pyridocarbazoles

Extensive studies of rigid dimers derived from three isomers of 7H-pyridocarbazole (with pyridine nitrogen in position 2, 3 or 4) and ellipticine (6H-pyridocarbazole) have shown that at physiological pH only the dimers quaternized on N_2 or N_3 by the rigid bis(ethylpiperidinyl) display binding affinities clearly larger (> 100 fold) than their monomeric precursors (Pelaprat *et al.*, 1980b). Moreover, within the compounds exhibiting high DNA affinity only those belonging to the series of 7H-pyrido[4,3-c]carbazole dimers elicit strong antitumour activity (see following section).

We assumed that such differences in the biological properties of these pyridocarbazole dimers should be due, at least partly, to the structures of their DNA intercalation complexes.

As was previously described (Krugh and Nuss, 1979), the structures of intercalation complexes can be investigated using autocomplementary oligonucleotides and measuring the changes in chemical shifts of drugs and base-pairs protons during their mutual interaction. At low concentration of oligonucleotides ($< 10^{-3}$M) and at room temperature, the concentration of base paired forms of autocomplementary ribodinucleosides such as CpG or GpC is very low (Krugh and Nuss, 1979). Addition of intercalating compounds such as the different monomeric pyridocarbazoles induces the formation of intercalated minihelixes stabilized by the Watson-Crick hydrogen bonding scheme.

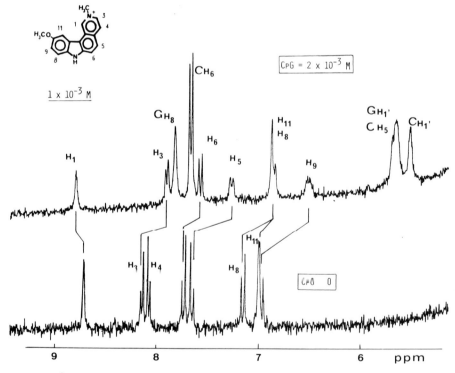

FIG. 4 ^{1}H NMR spectra of the aromatic part of 2-methyl-10-methoxy-7H-pyrido[4,3-c]carbazolium iodide 10^{-3}M performed at 270 MHz in deuteroacetate buffer, 5×10^{-3}M, pH 5.5, temp 25°C. Bottom, without CpG; top, in presence of CpG (2.2×10^{-3}M). The lines connecting the two spectra illustrate the differential shielding undergone by the pyridocarbazole aromatic protons.

As illustrated in Fig. 4 for the interaction of 2-methyl-10-methoxy-7H-pyrido[4,3-c]carbazolium iodide with the ribodinucleoside CpG, such a process induces a large shielding of the drug aromatic protons. These up-field shifts are due to the ring current effects of the super-imposed hydrogen-bonded base-pairs surrounding the intercalated pyridocarbazole. The stoichiometry of the complex can be obtained from a plot of the chemical shift of the drug proton NMR signal as a function of the concentration of the dinucleotide. The shape of the titration curve indicates a stoichiometry of approximately two CpG nucleosides for one pyridocarbazole. Furthermore it must be noticed that for monocationic drugs such as 2-methyl-10-methoxy-7H-pyrido-[4,3-c]carbazolium and 2-methyl 9-methoxy ellipticinium iodides complexes of 2-2, CpG-drug stoichiometries crystallize during NMR experiments. Such complexes correspond to a neutralization of the two phosphate groups of the dinucleoside by both a positively charged inter-calated drug and an additional one, stacked on the base pair of the minihelix.

As for most of the intercalating agents, all the studied pyrido-carbazoles interact preferentially with autocomplementary dinucleosides of 3'-5'-pyrimidine–purine sequence (Gaugain *et al.*, 1981).

Proposed geometries of intercalated complexes between CpG and pyridocarbazoles
Titration curves of the different pyridocarbazoles with CpG show that, in the minihelical complexes, the shielding of the ring protons is not identical. Therefore a geometry for the intercalating complex can be estimated with a good approximation using as described (Gaugain *et al.*, 1981; Laugâa *et al.*, 1981; Laugâa *et al.*, 1983):

1) the differences between the chemical shifts of the aromatic protons at infinite dilution and in the presence of an excess of autocomplementary dinucleoside,
2) the ring current and anisotropic effects of guanine and cytosine previously computed by Giessner-Prettre and Pullman (Giessner-Prettre and Pullman, 1976).

The geometries proposed for the intercalation of 2-methyl 9-methoxy ellipticinium iodide and 2-methyl 10-methoxy 7H-pyrido[4,3-c]carba-zolium iodide with CpG are reported in Fig. 5.

For the proposed complexes, the agreement between experimental induced shielding and computed values is within ± 10%. As shown in Fig. 5 the complex between CpG and the ellipticinium iodide is characterized by an orientation of the nitrogen of the pyrole ring towards

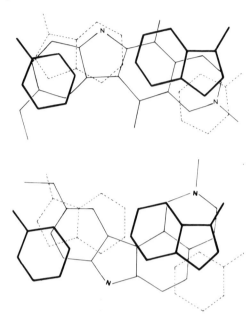

FIG. 5   Proposed intercalating geometries for 2-methyl-9-methoxyellipticinium iodide (top) and 2-methyl-10-methoxy-7H-pyrido[4,3-c]carbazolium iodide (bottom) with CpG, deduced from comparison of experimental and computed upfield shifts of drug aromatic protons (see text). Redrawing from Laugâa *et al.*, 1981.

the small groove and by a base turn angle, B = 18°, similar to that found at the DNA level (Tsai *et al.*, 1977).

This computed structure is quite similar to that found in the crystal of iodo-CpG-ellipticinium (Jain *et al.*, 1979) with the quaternized pyridine nitrogen located near the ribose–phosphate backbone. In the case of the 7H-pyridocarbazoles, the proposed geometry of the inter-calated minihelical complex is very different. Indeed, the pyrole nitrogen is now oriented towards the large groove and the positively charged *N*-methyl group is not sterically hindered in contrast to its situation in the CpG-ellipticinium complex (Laugâa *et al.*, 1981).

Therefore, in the bis-7H-pyridocarbazoles, the introduction of a spacer link on the pyridine nitrogen (especially on the N_2 position) may not modify greatly the orientation of the whole aromatic ring into the minihelix. On the other hand, a change of the geometry of inter-calation is required for bis-ellipticium. Assuming that the orientation of some substituent (for instance the 5 or 11 methyl group) with respect to the superimposed base pairs may play a major role in antitumour properties, the changes in the structure of DNA complexes imposed by dimerization of ellipticines could explain the loss of activity in the derived dimers (Pelaprat *et al.*, 1980b).

Antitumour Properties of 7H-Pyridocarbazole Dimers

L 1210 murine leukaemia was used for antitumour evaluation because of its good predictive value for activity in human cancer. The results are reported in Table 2 and compared with antitumour potency of doxorubicin and daunorubicin determined under strictly the same conditions. In the first instance, it can be noticed that two dimers 3 and 4 belonging to the 7H-pyrido[4,3-c]carbazolium series exhibit a strong antitumour activity whereas their monomeric precursors bearing an ethylpiperidine quaternizing chain are either completely inactive or very slightly active (Pelaprat *et al.*, 1980a).

TABLE 2

Comparison of the antitumour properties of rigid dimers from 7H-pyrido[4,3-c]carbazole and doxorubicin or daunorubicin

Tumour	Treatment	Dimer 3		Dimer 4		Doxorubicin		Daunorubicin	
		D.O. mg/kg	T/C %	D.O. mg/kg	T/C %	D.O. mg/kg	T/C %	D.O. mg/kg	T/C %
L 1210	one day	25	224 (2/9)	10	259 (1/10)	10	325 (5/10)	5	172 (1/10)
i.p.	day: + 1,5,9,13	6.25	212 (1/10)	5	241	5	288 (2/9)	2.5	179 (1/10)
B 16	one day	5	121	5	140	–	–	–	–
i.p.	day: + 1,4,7,9,11	–	–	5	142	–	–	–	–
Lewis	one day	5	0.54	2.5	0.54	–	–	–	–
i.p.	day: + 1,5,9,13	1.25	0.75	1.25	0.75	–	–	–	–

The values in brackets represent the number of survivors out of the total of treated animals

Obviously the linking chain (1,1'-bis-[N,N-dimethylamino ethyl]-4,4'-bipiperidine) by itself is inactive. Furthermore a substantial percentage of cured animals is obtained with 3 and the potency of the two dimers is of the same order as that of daunorubicin. It is interesting to observe on cultures of L 1210 the lack of cross-resistance between pyridocarbazole monomers (including ellipticines) and the active dimers. This strongly suggests that the mechanism of action of these latter compounds is different from that of their monomeric precursors and therefore that bis-intercalators represent a new class of antitumour agents.

In addition, the therapeutic index of these dimers is remarkably high since at doses corresponding to one fiftieth of the maximum sublethal dose a significant antitumour effect is still observed (Roques *et al.*, 1979a; Pelaprat *et al.*, 1980b).

Finally the most potent pyridocarbazole dimers display interesting antitumour activities both on the Lewis lung tumour and the B 16 melanoma. All these results obtained in the laboratory of J.B. Le Pecq, were confirmed by corresponding assays performed both in Rhône-Poulenc and N.C.I. Laboratories. One of these compounds prepared in large quantity by Roger Bellon Laboratory is now under clinical trial.

In conclusion the main objective of this project was to obtain anti-tumour agents by preparing dimeric intercalating compounds of high affinity for DNA.

Intercalation alone is not sufficient for biological activity and probably has to be accompanied by lethal modification induced in the DNA helix. Nevertheless, as shown with pyridocarbazole dimers, the probability of finding active derivatives is much higher among compounds exhibiting high affinity for DNA.

The topological concept of DNA-bis-intercalation started in 1975 with acridine dimers (Le Pecq *et al.*, 1975; Barbet *et al.*, 1975) whereas at the same time Waring and Wakelin reported the DNA bis-inter-calating property of "echinomycin" a natural antibiotic made up of two quinoline rings bridged by a cyclic peptide (Waring and Wakelin, 1974). Since these preliminary studies, an increasing number of laboratories has launched into the synthesis of potential DNA bis-intercalators and several of them exhibit interesting antitumour properties (Cain *et al.*, 1978; Kuhlman and Mosher, 1981).

Rational Design of Selective Effectors for μ and δ Opiate Receptors

Morphine and related drugs have been used for a long time as highly potent analgesics. However all these compounds display very undesirable side-effects such as respiratory depression, tolerance and dependence. Therefore, a considerable number of synthetic analgesics have been designed with the aim of eliminating or at least reducing these side-effects. Nevertheless, at this time, there is no potent analgesic which does not induce a physical dependence after chronic administration.

However, it seems that a gleam of hope for a rational approach to solve this challenging problem could arise from the differentiation of opiate binding-sites. Using morphine, benzomorphan and N-allyl-norphenazocine, Martin *et al.* (1976) observed in spinal dogs various pharmacological responses that they interpreted in terms of three kinds of opiate receptors μ, $\varkappa$ and σ. So, morphine and structurally related compounds would interact with μ-receptors to elicit analgesia and euphoria whereas benzomorphans such as ethylketocyclazocine would bind preferentially to $\varkappa$-receptors producing sedative effects and weak antinociceptive responses without strong dependence. The σ-receptors could correspond to the binding site of phencyclidine and analogues in accordance with the similar psychotic effects elicited by these drugs and *N*-allylnorphenazocine.

The occurrence of heterogeneity of opiate receptor subtypes in the central nervous system was strongly confirmed by the discovery of several brain peptides which could behave as endogenous agonists (Hughes *et al.*, 1975; Lord *et al.*, 1977; Chang *et al.*, 1979; Cavkin *et al.*, 1982). The characterization of these receptor subtypes and the development of highly selective effectors could represent a new approach to the resolution of the various effects elicited by classical narcotics.

Heterogeneity of Opioid Peptides and Receptors

The two pentapeptides Met-enkephalin, Tyr-Gly-Gly-Phe-Met and Leu-enkephalin are now considered as classical neurotransmitters or neuro-modulators since they are localized in specific neurones, released by nociceptive stimuli and degraded by specific enzymes. Moreover, implication of enkephalins in analgesia was clearly demonstrated by the naloxone reversible analgesic effect of Thiorphan (Roques *et al.*, 1980b), a selective inhibitor of the enkephalin degrading enzyme "enkephalinase" (Malfroy *et al.*, 1978).

On the other hand the enkephalins interact with at least two distinct binding sites: a high affinity site or δ-receptor ($K_D = 0.5-2\,nM$) which displays a high specificity for peptide-structures and a lower affinity site or μ-receptor ($K_D = 5-10\,nM$) which recognizes preferentially more rigid structure such as morphine and derivatives. The distribution of these binding sites is heterogenous since δ-sites are more abundant in the limbic-system whereas μ-sites are more concentrated in periac-queducal grey matter. Likewise a large receptor heterogeneity occurs in peripheral organs since the guinea pig ileum (GPI), the mouse vas deferens (MVD) and the rabbit vas deferens can be respectively considered as models of peripheral μ, δ and ϰ receptors. This is clearly evidenced in Table 3, from the inhibition of electrically stimulated organs by morphine, Leu-enkephalin and ethylketocyclazocine which behave respectively as relatively selective agonists of μ, δ and ϰ receptors.

Therefore, all the results support the classification of Martin *et al.* (1976) although a new binding site (δ-receptor) has to be added to those proposed by these authors. The parmacological relevance of this receptor-heterogeneity is supported by observations such as: lack of cross-tolerance between μ and δ ligands; difference in the ontogenesis of μ and δ receptors; autoradiographic measurements in brain. It remains

TABLE 3

Inhibitory potency of Leu-enkephalin, morphine and ethylketocyclazocine on electrically stimulated contractions of guinea-pig ileum (GPI), mouse was deferens (MVD) and rabbit was deferens (RVD). The values are the mean of at least 15 different experiments (SD < ± 10%).

	IC_{50} (nM)		
	GPI (μ)	MVD (δ)	RVD ($\varkappa$)
Leu-enkephalin	395	8.2	> 10 000
Morphine	70	490.0	> 1 000
Ethylketocyclazocine	0.5	4.5	46

however to firmly establish:

1) the pharmacological responses elicited by selective μ, δ or $\varkappa$ receptor stimulation,
2) that each binding site is a distinct entity, rather than each affecting a common opiate regulator by allosteric coupling,
3) the nature of the biological transduction sites (cyclase or ion channel) associated with each putative receptor (review in Roques *et al.*, 1982 and Wood, 1982).

Obviously, unambiguous answers to these questions require highly selective ligands for each receptor-subtype.

Rational Design of Highly Specific μ and δ Agonists

In 1976, using NMR spectroscopy, we demonstrated structural analogies between a morphine derivative belonging to the class of oripavines and Met or Leu-eukephalin in their preferential conformation (Roques *et al.*, 1976c). So the spatial disposition of the tyramine moiety which is crucial for receptor binding is similar in the alkaloid and the peptide.

Moreover the oripavine molecule contains an additional phenyl ring which mimics the Phe[4] side chain of enkephalins. Taking into account that most narcotics are devoid of such an additional phenyl residue we thought that this moiety could be the crucial component for selective δ-recognition. This hypothesis was checked by replacing this aromatic ring with several hydrophobic aliphatic side chains (Roques *et al.*, 1979b).

Extensive conformational studies performed by NMR (Garbay-Jaureguiberry *et al.*, 1977; Roques *et al.*, 1980a; Garbay-Jaureguiberry *et al.*, 1982) and theoretical computations (Maigret *et al.*, 1981) allowed the demonstration that μ-specific binding requires short peptides with highly folded conformations containing a lipophilic D-amino acid in position 2. This is illustrated in Table 4 by the good selectivity of TRIMU 5 which is more potent on the μ-receptors of GPI than on the δ-sites of MVD.

TABLE 4

Inhibitory potency of modified enkephalins on the electrically stimulated contractions of guinea-pig ileum (GPI) and mouse vas deferens (MVD). The values are the mean $\pm$ SEM of at least five independent experiments with Met-E as internal standard in each assay. The ratio of $IC_{50}GPI/IC_{50}MVD$ defines the μ/δ selectivity factor of a given compound.

Compounds	GPI (IC_{50} nM)	MVD (IC_{50} nM)	$\dfrac{IC_{50} \text{ GPI}}{IC_{50} \text{ MVD}}$
Tyr-Gly-Gly-Phe-Met	200 ± 19	13 ± 1.5	15.38
Tyr-D.Ala-Gly-NHCH-CH$_2$CH(CH$_3$)$_2$ (TRIMU 4) CH$_3$	263 ± 28	1133 ± 90	0.23
Tyr-D.Ala-Gly-NH(CH$_2$)$_2$-CH(CH$_3$)$_2$ (TRIMU 5)	359 ± 73	3694 ± 320	0.09
Tyr-NHCH-CO-Gly-NHCH-CH$_2$-CH(CH$_3$)$_2$ CH$_3$ CH$_3$	5100 ± 380	0.40	
Tyr-D.Ala-Gly-N-CH-CH$_2$-CH(CH$_3$)$_2$ Et CH$_3$	239 ± 15	1950 ± 40	0.12
Tyr-D.Ser-Gly-NHCH-CH$_2$-CH(CH$_3$)$_2$ (TRIMU 6) CH$_3$	797 ± 40	1073 ± 160	0.75
Tyr-D.Ala-Gly(Me)Phe-NH(CH$_2$)$_2$OH (DAGO)	13 ± 0.50	83 ± 7	0.15

Starting from these results highly selective δ-ligands were developed. So the replacement in the Tyr-D-Ala-Gly-Phe-D-Leu, DADLE (a peptide commonly used as a δ-specific probe) of D-Ala^2 by a hydrophilic amino acid such as D-Ser^2 led to an increase in δ-selectivity by adverse recognition of the corresponding μ-receptor hydrophobic subsite. A definitive increase in δ-specificity was obtained by lengthening the peptide sequence through addition of a sixth hydrophilic amino acid which inhibits the folding tendency of the peptide. So DSLET and DTLET are respectively about 1000 fold and 3000 fold more potent on MVD (δ-receptors) than on GPI (μ-receptors) (Table 5). The crucial role of the aromatic Phe^4 residue in δ-receptor recognition is clearly shown by the strongly decreased δ-affinity elicited by replacement of Phe^4 in DSLET by Leu^4. All these results allowed us to propose a structural model for selective μ or δ-recognition (Fournié-Zaluski *et al.*, 1981).

Binding Characteristics of Selective μ and δ Ligands

The results obtained on peripheral tissue were extended to the brain receptor level. For such a purpose the most selective ligands DAGO,

TABLE 5

Relationships between the sequence of modified enkephalins and their selectivity for
μ or δ opiate-receptors. The experiments were performed as described in Table 4.

Compounds	GPI		MVD		IC_{50} GPI
	IC_{50} (nM)	Rel.pot.	IC_{50} (nM)	Rel.pot.	IC_{50} MVD
Tyr-Gly-Gly-Phe-Met	200 ± 19	1.00	13.00 ± 1.5	1.0	15.38
Tyr-D.Ala-Gly-Phe-D.Leu (DADLE)	48 ± 5	4.16	0.55 ± 0.09	23.6	87.30
Tyr-D.Ser-Gly-Phe-D.Leu	140 ± 20	1.43	0.85 ± 0.1	15.3	164.7
Tyr-D.Ser-Gly-Phe-Leu-Thr (DSLET)	406 ± 30	0.49	0.40 ± 0.1	32.5	1015.0
Tyr-D.Thr-Gly-Phe-Leu-Thr (DTLET)	460 ± 60	0.43	0.15 ± 0.012	86.6	3067.0
Tyr-D.Ser-Gly-Leu-Leu-Thr	$2,000 \pm 120$	0.10	$3,060 \pm 400$	0.004	0.65

DSLET and DTLET were tritiated and their binding characteristics were
investigated on a synaptosomal fraction of crude rat brain (David *et
al.*, 1982; Zajac *et al.*, 1983). The μ-selective ligand [^{3}H]DAGO interacts with only one class of sites ($K_D = 3.8$ nM, $B_{max} = 0.19$ pmol/mg)
whereas under the same conditions [^{3}H] DADLE binds to both μ and
δ receptor subtypes with $K_D = 2$ nM, $B_{max} = 0.10$ pmole/mg and $K_D =
20$ nM, $B_{max} = 0.20$ pmole/mg, respectively.

In contrast to this latter peptide, [^{3}H] DSLET and [^{3}H] DTLET
interact with only one class of binding sites (δ-receptors) with DTLET
showing an interesting high affinity. The factor of selectivity was
estimated in competition experiments from the ratio of K_IDAGO
(μ)/K_I DSLET (δ-receptors). DSLET and DTLET are considered, at
this time, as the most potent and selective ligands for δ-receptors.
Moreover these peptides, as well as DAGO, do not recognize $\varkappa$-receptors
as shown by their $IC_{50} > 1000$ nM. Finally the pharmacological profile
of the dimeric tetrapeptide [Tyr-D-Ala-Gly-Phe-NH(CH$_2$)$_6$]$_2$, recently
claimed (Shimohigashi *et al.*, 1982) to be a superior δ-probe from
binding studies on different preparation, is clearly less favourable than
those of DSLET and DTLET (Table 6).

Pharmacological Characterization of μ and δ Binding Sites

Owing to the strong dissociation between μ and δ recognition of DAGO,
DSLET and DTLET, the 50 times better analgesic effects of DAGO
as compared to the δ-hexapeptides demonstrate the preferential involvement of μ-receptors in analgesia (Gacel *et al.*, 1981). Moreover, there
is no potentiation of the effects of subanalgesic doses of DAGO by
DTLET and conversely. This indicates that the recently proposed

TABLE 6

Selectivity of modified enekphalins on crude rat brain membranes (with [^{3}H]DAGO, 1 nM and [^{3}H]DSLET, 2 nM as respective μ and δ ligands).

Compounds	K_I (nM)		K_I DSLET
	[^{3}H] DAGO	[^{3}H] DSLET	K_I DAGO
Tyr-D-Ala-Gly-MePhe-Gly-ol (DAGO)	3.90 ± 0.80	700.00 ± 95.00	179.0
Tyr-D-Ala-Gly-Phe-D-Leu (DADLE)	7.70 ± 1.10	2.40 ± 0.31	0.31
Tyr-D-Ser-Gly-Phe-Leu-Thr (DSLET)	31.00 ± 5.00	4.80 ± 0.80	0.15
Tyr-D-Thr-Gly-Phe-Leu-Thr (DTLET)	25.30 ± 2.50	1.35 ± 0.15	0.053
Tyr-D-Ala-Gly-Phe-NH ($\overset{\mid}{C}$H$_2$)$_{12}$ Tyr-D-Ala-Gly-Phe-NH	43.00 ± 7.70	11.50 ± 4.30	0.27

In binding experiments, the K_I values are the means of five independent determinations and are obtained assuming competitive inhibition from computer analysis of Hill plots.

allosteric coupling between μ and δ binding sites is not observed *in vivo* using highly selective ligands. The same negative results occur when the endogenous peptides are protected from metabolic degradation by bestatin (aminopeptidase inhibitor) and thiorphan (enkephalinase inhibitor) (Roques *et al.*, 1980b).

It seems therefore that pain regulation preferentially involves μ-receptor stimulation (Chaillet *et al.*, 1983). However the pharmacological role of the δ-receptor remains unclear although some experiments seem to indicate its implication in behavioural responses (Righter *et al.*, 1980; Belluzzi and Stein, 1977). Along these lines, the first unambiguous distinction between the pharmacological responses elicited by selective μ or δ receptor stimulation arises from *in vivo* and *in vitro* experiments on dopamine release. Indeed it was shown that opiate receptors (probably presynaptic) occur along the nigrostriatal pathway.

Using the push-pull cannula method, a large increase in dopamine release was observed after administration of DSLET. Such an effect, which was hardly antagonized by the μ-antagonist naloxone, was not obtained with TRIMU 4, a specific μ-agonist. This effect was clearly confirmed by *in vitro* experiments using striatal slices. As shown in Fig. 6, the release of [^{3}H] dopamine from slices pre-incubated with [^{3}H] tyrosine is strongly increased by DSLET whereas TRIMU 4 and morphine are unable to produce this effect (Chesselet *et al.*, 1981; Chesselet *et al.*, 1982).

The occurrence of physiological regulation of dopamine release in the nigrostriatal pathway through δ-selective stimulation is of considerable interest because of the probable malfunctioning of dopamine

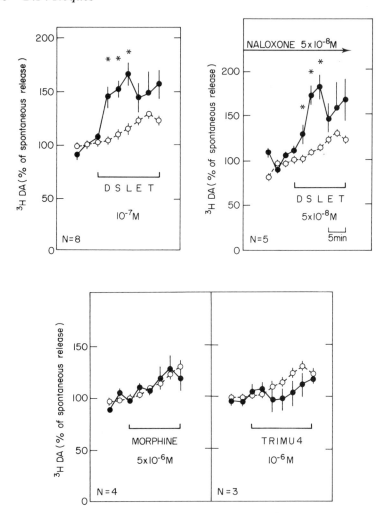

FIG. 6   Effects of μ (TRIMU 4) and δ (DSLET) agonists on the ^{3}H dopamine release from rat striatal slices (Chesselet *et al.*, 1981; Chesselet *et al.*, 1982). The ^{3}H-dopamine (^{3}H DA) is synthesized from the ^{3}H-tyrosine present in the pre-incubation medium. The results are expressed in % of the ^{3}H-DA release in the absence of agonist. Each point corresponds to the mean ± SEM of 6 different experiments. The horizontal bars indicate the period of administration of the agonist.

neurones in various mental illnesses and Parkinson disease. Our knowledge of the role of δ-receptors will increase in the next few years owing to the synthesis of selective antagonists such as *N,N*-diallyl-Tyr-Gly-ψ(CH$_2$S)-Phe-Leu, ICI 154,129 (Gormley *et al.*, 1982). The first pharmacological assays with this compound seem to confirm the implication of δ-receptor subtypes in behavioural responses (Gormley *et al.*, 1982).

Future Aspects of Drug Design in the Field of Opioid Peptides

The discovery of enkephalins has not led as expected to the immediate design of potent analgesics devoid of dependence effects. This has been partly due to the fact that in the initial synthetic approaches the occurrence of multiple receptors was not taken into account. Along these lines, it is very interesting to note that compounds eliciting a reduced withdrawal syndrome such as some benzomorphans and the recently clinically investigated opioid peptide metkephamid (Calimlim *et al.*, 1982) interact preferentially with $\varkappa$- or δ-receptors (or both) rather than on μ-binding sites. Since it has been observed that several opioid peptides such as Met and Leu-enkephalin, the $\varkappa$-agonist dynorphin, Met-E-Arg-Gly-Leu and others are released from larger precursors it is apparent that the system of pain-regulation, and the reward system, probably involve a number of peptides interacting selectively with specific receptors. Therefore, investigation of the metabolism of these precursors and of the opioid peptides as well as the design of highly selective agonists or antagonists offer exciting new approaches to the design of new analgesics and psychoactive agents.

Using such a rational approach we have recently prepared thiorphan (Roques *et al.*, 1980b) and retro-thiorphan (Roques *et al.*, 1983) which behave as highly potent and selective inhibitors of the Gly^3-Phe^4 enkephalin cleaving enzyme. As expected these compounds display naloxone reversible analgesic properties. Preliminary experiments seem to indicate that these inhibitors do not induce significant tolerance and dependence effects after chronic administration in animals.

Acknowledgements

This work has been supported by grants from DGRST, Fondation pour la Recherche Médicale Française, Association pour le Développement de la Recherche sur le Cancer, Roger Bellon and Rhône-Poulenc Laboratories.

Mrs Annick Bouju is gratefully acknowledged for her excellent technical assistance in the preparation of the manuscript.

Most of the results presented in this paper arise from studies performed in our laboratory (ERA 613 CNRS, SC 21 INSERM) and the laboratories of J.B. le Pecq and J. Costentin (Université de Rouen). All the co-authors of these studies are gratefully acknowledged.

References

Barbet, J., Roques, B.P. and Le Pecq, J.B. (1975). *C.R. Acad. Sci., Série D* **281**, 851–853.

Barbet, J., Roques, B.P., Combrisson, S. and Le Pecq, J.B. (1976). *Biochemistry* **15**, 2642–2650.

Bauer, W. and Vinograd, J. (1970). *J. Mol. Biol.* **47**, 419–435.

Belluzi, J.D. and Stein, L. (1977). *Nature (London)* **266**, 556–558.

Butour, J.L., Delain, E., Coulaud, D., Le Pecq, J.B., Barbet, J. and Roques, B.P. (1978). *Biopolymers* **17**, 873–886.

Cain, B.F., Baguley, B.C. and Denny, W.A. (1978). *J. Med. Chem.* **21**, 658–668.

Calimlim, J.F., Wardell, W.M., Lasagna, L. and Cos, C. (1982). *Lancet* **19**, 1374–1376.

Capelle, N., Barbet, J., Dessen, P., Blanquet, S., Roques, B.P. and Le Pecq, J.B. (1979). *Biochemistry* **15**, 3354–3362.

Cavkin, C., James, I.F. and Goldstein, A. (1982). *Science* **215**, 413–415.

Chaillet, P., Marçais-Collado, H., Costentin, J., Zajac, J.M., Gacel, G. and Roques, B.P. (1983). *Life Sci.*, submitted.

Chang, K.J., Cooper, B.R., Hazum, E. and Cuatrecasas, P. (1979). *Mol. Pharmacol.* **16**, 91–104.

Chesselet, M.F., Cheramy, A., Reisine, T.D. and Glowinski, J. (1981). *Nature (London)* **291**, 320–322.

Chesselet, M.F., Cheramy, A., Reisine, T.D., Lubetzki, C., Glowinski, J., Fournié-Zaluski, M.C. and Roques, B.P. (1982). *Life Sci.* **31**, 2420–2424.

David, M., Moisand, C., Meunier, J.C., Morgat, J.L., Gacel, G. and Roques, B.P. (1982). *Eur. J. Pharmacol.* **78**, 385–387.

Delbarre, A., Roques, B.P. and Le Pecq, J.B. (1977). *C.R. Acad. Sci. Sér D* **284**, 81–84.

Delbarre, A., Gaugain, B., Markovits, J., Vilar, A., Le Pecq, J.B. and Roques, B.P. (1981). *In* "Proc. of the Jerusalem Symposia on Quantum Chemistry and Biochemistry, Intermolecular Forces" (B. Pullman, ed.), vol. 14, pp. 273–283. Reidel Publishing Company, Holland.

Dulbecco, R. (1982). *La Recherche* **13** (139), 1426–1436.

Fournié-Zaluski, M.C., Gacel, G., Maigret, B., Premilat, S. and Roques, B.P. (1981). *Mol. Pharmacol.* **20**, 484–491.

Gacel, G., Fournié-Zaluski, M.C., Fellion, E. and Roques, B.P. (1981). *J. Med. Chem.* **24**, 1119–1124.

Garbay-Jaureguiberry, C., Roques, B.P., Oberlin, R., Anteunis, M., Combrisson, S. and Lallemand, J.Y. (1977). *F.E.B.S. Lett.* **76**, 93.

Garbay-Jaureguiberry, C., Marion, D., Fellion, E. and Roques, B.P. (1982). *Int. J. Pept. Protein Res.* **20**, 443–450.

Gaugain, B., Barbet, J., Oberlin, R., Roques, B.P. and Le Pecq, J.B. (1978a). *Biochemistry* **17**, 5071–5078.

Gaugain, B., Barbet, J., Capelle, N., Roques, B.P. and Le Pecq, J.B. (1978b). *Biochemistry* **17**, 5078–5088.

Gaugain, B., Markovits, J., Le Pecq, J.B. and Roques, B.P. (1981). *Biochemistry* **20**, 3035–3042.

Giessner-Prettre, C. and Pullman, B. (1976). *Biochem. Biophys. Res. Commun.* **70** (2), 578–581.

Gormley, J.J., Morley, J.S., Priestley, T., Shaw, J.S., Turnbull, M.J. and Wheeler, H. (1982). *Life Sci.* **27**, 1263–1266.

Hugues, J., Smith, T.W., Kosterlitz, H.W., Fothergill, L.A., Morgan, B.A. and Morris, H.R. (1975). *Nature (London)* **258**, 577–579.

Jain, S.C., Bhan-Dary, K.K. and Sobell, H.M. (1979). *J. Mol. Biol.* **135**, 813–840.

Juret, P., Heron, J.F., Couette, J.F., Delozier, T. and Le Talaer, J.Y. (1982). *Cancer Treat. Rep.* **66** (11), 1909–1916.

Krugh, T.R. and Nuss, M.E. (1979). In "Biological Applications of Magnetic Resonance" (R.G. Shulman, ed.), pp. 113–176. Academic Press, New York.

Kuhlman, K.F. and Mosher, C.W. (1981). *J. Med. Chem.* **24**, 1333–1337.

Laugâa, P., Delbarre, A. and Roques, B.P. (1981). *Biochimie* **63**, 967–973.

Laugâa, P., Delbarre, A., Le Pecq, J.B. and Roques, B.P. (1983). *Eur. J. Biochem.* **134**, 163–173.

Le Pecq, J.B., Le Bret., M., Barbet, J. and Roques, B.P. (1975). *Proc. Natl. Acad. Sci.* **72**, 2915–2919.

Lerman, L.S. (1961). *J. Mol. Biol.* **3**, 18–30.

Lord, J.A.H., Waterfield, A.A., Hughes, J. and Kosterlitz, H.W. (1977). *Nature (London)* **267**, 495–499.

Maigret, B., Premilat, S., Fournié-Zaluski, M.C. and Roques, B.P. (1981). *Biochem. Biophys. Res. Commun.* **99**, 267–274.

Malfroy, B., Swerts, J.P., Guyon, A., Roques, B.P. and Schwartz, J.C. (1978). *Nature (London)* **276**, 523–526.

Markovits, J., Roques, B.P. and Le Pecq, J.B. (1979). *Anal. Biochem.* **94**, 259–264.

Markovits, J., Gaugain, B., Barbet, J., Roques, B.P., Le Pecq, J.B. (1981a). *Biochemistry* **20**, 3042–3048.

Markovits, J., Blanquet, S., Dessen, P., Roques, B.P. and Le Pecq. J.B. (1981b). *Biochem. Pharm.* **30**, 1557–1562.

Markovits, J., Gaugain, B., Roques, B.P. and Le Pecq, J.B. (1981c). In "Proceedings of the Jerusalem Symposia on Quantum Chemistry and Biochemistry, Intermolecular Forces (B. Pullman, ed.), vol. 14, pp. 285–298. Reidel Publishing Company, Holland.

Martin, W.R., Eades, C.G., Thompson, J.A., Huppler, R.E. and Gilbert, P.E. (1976). *J. Pharmacol. Exp. Ther.* **197**, 517–532.

Pelaprat, D., Oberlin, R., Le Guen, I., Le Pecq, J.B. and Roques, B.P. (1980a). *J. Med. Chem.* **23**, 1330–1335.

Pelaprat, D., Delbarre, A., Le Guen, I., Le Pecq, J.B. and Roques, B.P. (1980b). *J. Med. Chem.* **23**, 1336–1342.

Reinhardt, C.G., Roques, B.P. and Le Pecq, B.P. (1982). *Biochem. Biophys. Res. Commun.* **104** (4), 1376–1385.

Revet, B.M.J., Schmir, M. and Vinograd, J. (1971). *Nature (London) New Biol.* **229**, 10–13.

Righter, H., Jensen, R.A., Martinez, J.L., Messing, R.B., Wasquez, B.J., Liang, K.C. and Mc Gaugh, J.L. (1980). *Proc. Natl. Acad. Sci. USA* **77**, 2729–2732.

Roques, B.P., Barbet, J., Oberlin, R. and Le Pecq, J.B. (1976a). *C.R. Acad. Sci. Sér. D* **283**, 1355–1357.

Roques, B.P., Barbet, J. and Le Pecq, J.B. (1976b). *C.R. Acad. Sci. Sér D* **283**, 1453–1455.

Roques, B.P., Garbay-Jaureguiberry, C., Oberlin, R., Anteunis, M. and Lala, A.K. (1976c). *Nature (London)* **262**, 778–779.

Roques, B.P., Pelaprat, D., Le Guen, I., Porcher, G., Gosse, C. and Le Pecq, J.B. (1979a). *Biochem. Pharmacol.* **28**, 1811–1815.

Roques, B.P., Gacel, G., Fournié-Zaluski, M.C., Senault, B. and Lecomte, J.M. (1979b). *Eur. J. Pharmacol.* **60**, 109–110.

Roques, B.P., Garbay-Jaureguiberry, C., Bajusz, S., Maigret, B. (1980a). *Eur. J. Biochem.* **113**, 105–119.

Roques, B.P., Fournié-Zaluski, M.C., Soroca, E., Lecomte, J.M., Malfroy, B., Llorens, C. and Schwartz, J.C. (1980b). *Nature (London)* **288**, 286–288.

Roques, B.P., Fournié-Zaluski, M.C., Gacel, G., David, M., Meunier, J.C., Maigret, B. and Morgat, J.L. (1982). *Adv. Biochem. Psychopharmacol.* **33**, 321–331.

Roques, B.P., Lucas-Soroca, E., Chaillet, P., Costentin, J. and Fournie-Zaluski, M.C. (1983). *Proc. Natl. Acad. Sci.* **80**, 3178–3182.

Saucier, J.M., Festy, B. and Le Pecq, J.B. (1971). *Biochimie* **53**, 973–980.

Shimohigashi, Y., Costa, J., Chen, H. and Rodbard, D. (1982). *Nature (London)* **297**, 332–335.

Tsai, C.C., Jain, S.C. and Sobell, H.M. (1977). *J. Mol. Biol.* **114**, 301–315.

Waring, M. (1970). *J. Mol. Biol.* **54**, 247–279.

Waring, M.J. and Wakelin, L.P.G. (1974). *Nature (London)* **252**, 653–657.

Wood, P.L. (1982). *Neuropharmacology* **21**, 487–497.

Zajac, J.M., Gacel, G., Dodey, P., Morgat, J.L., Chaillet, P., Costentin, J. and Roques, B.P. (1983). *Biochem. Biophys. Res. Commun.* **111**, 390–397.

Discussion

Chairman: Professor Tomlinson

Professor Rabin
Are any of the modified enkephalins active on intravenous injection? One of the problems with the enkephalins, of course, is that they do not get into the brain. Are any of the compounds better than the existing known enkephalins?

Professor Roques
Experiments have been carried out by i.c.v. injection in order to eliminate the problem of pharmacokinetics. I think it is possible to obtain peptides which easily cross the blood–brain barrier and also enter the gastro-intestinal tract. It is a problem, but it can be overcome.

Recent studies performed in Rhône-Poulenc laboratories have clearly shown that DTLET and DAGO crosses the blood–brain barrier after i.v. injection. Thus behavioural effects are evident at a dose ~ 5 mg/kg in mice. Moverover it must observed that a synthetic opioid peptide like Tyr-D-Ala-Gly-(Me)Phe-Met(0)-ol (Sandoz FK 33-824) is about five times more active than morphine as an analgesic after oral administration

Professor Stevens
What evidence do you have to show that bis-intercalation has anything to do with antitumour activity? Does the fact that these compounds bis-intercalate correlate with antitumour activity? Are you not impressed by the compelling evidence to suggest that compounds of this type exert their activity outside the cell rather than inside the nucleus?

Professor Roques
We are uncertain about the first two questions. My hypothesis is that there is a relationship. DNA is the target for compounds such as intercalating agents and intercalation with DNA produces a cytotoxic effect, killing the cancer cells and, unfortunately other cells. Bis-intercalators have a very high affinity as compared with the monomers, which are completely inactive. This is the first point. The second point is that the active bis-intercalators do not cross-react with their parent monomers, or with daunorubicin, adriamycin and other kinds of substance. It is an interesting result.

8 The Design and Medicinal Applications of Transition State Analogues

P.R. ANDREWS and D.A. WINKLER

School of Pharmaceutical Chemistry, Victorian College of Pharmacy Ltd., 381 Royal Parade, Parkville, Victoria 3052, Australia

Introduction

Increased understanding of enzyme structure and mechanism has led to the development of several rational approaches to the design of potent enzyme inhibitors. These include active site directed irreversible inhibitors (Baker, 1967), mechanism-based irreversible inhibitors (Rando, 1974) and transition state analogues.

The basis for the transition state analogue approach was first suggested by Pauling (1946), who speculated that the catalytic specificity of enzymes required the active site of the enzyme and the transition state of the catalysed reaction to be structurally complementary. Molecules which resembled the transition state structure could thus be expected to bind the active site much more tightly than the natural substrate. This concept was taken up and elaborated by Lienhard (1972, 1973) and by Wolfenden (1969, 1972, 1976), whose work catalysed the subsequent development of several therapeutically interesting transition state analogues.

In this chapter we shall describe the steps involved in the design of transition state analogues, and then review some of their major areas of current and potential therapeutic significance. We shall also endeavour to provide a critical appraisal of the transition state analogue approach as an alternative pathway to novel drugs.

DRUG DESIGN: FACT OR FANTASY
ISBN 0.12.388180.3

Steps in Transition State Analogue Design

The process of transition state analogue design may be conveniently divided into the following steps (Andrews, 1979; Brodbeck, 1981)

1) Select an appropriate enzyme catalysed reaction as the target for inhibition.
2) Determine the mechanism of action of the selected enzyme.
3) Define the likely transition state structure(s).
4) Identify chemically stable analogues of the transition state(s).

Of these four steps only the first can normally be completed unequivocally, and a number of options are available at each stage. Some of these are discussed below.

Selection of Target Enzyme

The general principles governing the choice of target enzyme (Albert, 1979) apply equally to transition state analogues and other enzyme inhibitors. It should be noted, however, that selective inhibition of the "same" enzyme from different species cannot be expected from transition state analogues, since transition state binding ability is the *least* likely feature to vary from one species to another. Selective toxicity must therefore be sought either at the pharmacokinetic level or by choosing an enzyme that is essential only to the target species or tissue.

Single substrate or multisubstrate?

The nature of the substrate(s) is an important factor in the choice of target enzyme. Reactions involving a single small substrate molecule have the advantage that the transition state structure can often be tightly defined, but they suffer from the disadvantage that relatively few binding groups are available for specifying the inhibitory activity. Multisubstrate reactions, on the other hand, have transition states with many potential binding groups, but the relative orientations of the substrates in the transition state are much more difficult to define. Further difficulties arise if the architecture of the enzyme requires the substrates to enter the active site from different directions, in which case a multisubstrate analogue may not be able to gain access to its potential binding site. The crystal structure of dihydrofolate reductase (Matthews *et al.*, 1978), for example, suggests that the channel connecting the dihydrofolate and NADPH binding sites is probably too narrow to allow the passage of either molecule.

Reactions involving a single large substrate, such as a peptide, combine many of the advantages of single and multisubstrate reactions, but the greater flexibility of these molecules means that the transition state conformation is hard to define. It may thus be difficult to take advantage of the extra binding groups in the design of analogues.

Determination of Enzyme Mechanism

Information on the structure and mechanism of the target enzyme is a valuable aid in both the determination of transition state structures and the design of likely analogues. Even in the absence of specific information on the target enzyme it is often possible to extrapolate from data on related enzymes. The compilations of Walsh (1979) and Bernstein *et al.* (1977) are useful sources of mechanistic and structural information, respectively.

Definition of Transition State Structures

Because transition states exist only fleetingly it is not possible to make a direct experimental determination of their structures. Isotope effects provide some indirect information, and these and other techniques have recently been reviewed (Gandour and Schowen, 1978).

In the absence of experimental data the likely structure of the transition state is frequently estimated by chemical intuition. Such estimates are really based on the accepted rules of organic reaction mechanisms, and are more likely to approximate metastable intermediates than high energy transition state structures. The intuitive approach has nevertheless proved successful in a number of cases, and will no doubt continue to be favoured by many medicinal chemists.

Within the last few years, with the development of high speed computers, it has become feasible to use quantum mechanical methods as an alternative to the intuitive method (Jug, 1980). The quantum mechanical methods available can be broadly classified as "semi-empirical" and *ab initio*. The choice of a molecular orbital technique to be applied to any particular transition state problem depends primarily on how simple a chemical model can reasonably be used to represent the reaction. In most enzyme catalysed reaction mechanisms, the computer time required for geometry optimizing *ab initio* calculations is prohibitive, and semi-empirical techniques must be used.

The semi-empirical methods which have been applied most frequently to transition state studies are MINDO/3 (Bingham *et al.*, 1975), MNDO (Dewar and Thiel, 1977) and PRDDO (Halgren and Lipscomb, 1973). Of these, MINDO/3 provides satisfactory activation energies and apparently reasonable transition state geometries, although it gives an inadequate description of some hydrogen transfer reactions (Scheiner,

1980); MNDO is better in this respect. PRDDO may be the semi-empirical method of choice (Scheiner, 1980), although it has not yet been widely tested. *Ab initio* calculations should give the best representation of transition state structures (Maggiora and Christoffersen, 1978), although they may fail if too small a basis set is used (Dedieu and Veillard, 1970).

There are three main ways in which the structure of the transition state of a chemical reaction may be determined using the quantum mechanical techniques discussed above.

Brute force method   This is conceptually the simplest technique, involving the computation of the complete potential energy surface and the location of the transition state by inspection. Unfortunately this technique rapidly becomes untenable, even for a moderately sized molecule, due to the large numbers of degrees of freedom involved.

Minimum energy path approach   This method involves the selection of an appropriate *independent variable* which is well behaved over the entire course of the reaction. This may be a bond length, bond angle or internuclear distance, and should be a monotonically increasing or decreasing function of sufficient range over the entire reaction path to ensure an adequate description of the extent of reaction. The procedure then involves the determination of the minimum energy path produced by varying the independent variable in fixed (usually uniform) steps and minimizing the total energy of the system with respect to the remaining variables.

This approach suffers from the disadvantage that it is easy to miss the transition state by poor choice of independent variable or step size. Examples of the dangers of constrained minimization are discussed by McIver and Komornicki (1972) and Dewar and Kirschner (1971a, b, 1974).

Direct determination of transition states   In order to overcome the above difficulties, attempts have been made to determine transition state structures directly, using a nonlinear search of the potential surface for points which satisfy the appropriate mathematical conditions for transition states. Murrell and Laidler (1968) have shown that for a saddle or col point corresponding to a transition state, there will be one and only one negative eigenvalue of the force constant matrix. The eigenvector corresponding to this eigenvalue is called the *transition vector*. Backward or forward movement along the transition vector with subsequent geometry optimization will lead to the reactant or product geometries.

The location of the stationary points can be determined numerically by a number of techniques. The first of these was proposed by McIver and Komornicki (1972) and involves minimizing the gradient norm using nonlinear search techniques. The problem with this technique is that it locates all extremum points, and force constant matrices must be calculated to determine whether they are minima, maxima, inflection points or saddle points.

Recently, this technique has been improved by Schlegel (1982) and Spangler *et al.* (1982). The calculations are done in a manner which constrains the force constant matrix to contain only one negative eigenvalue, the eigenvectors of which define a path to the transition state. The programs can thus locate transition states exclusively, and ignore minima and maxima.

Calculate or estimate?
As is evident from the preceding discussion a full calculation of the transition state structure can be very time-consuming. Is it really worthwhile, or is chemical intuition enough?

We tend to favour a dual approach. The intuitive estimate provides a very rapid initial transition state structure and some approximate analogues. Synthesis and testing of these analogues can thus be proceeding at the same time as molecular orbital calculations, and may provide valuable feedback to the next phase of analogue design. Calculations, on the other hand, produce detailed transition state geometries as well as extra insight into the mechanisms of enzymatic catalysis and inhibition.

The ideal solution may eventually be a combination of both approaches. Thus, a library of rigorous *ab initio* calculations defining the electronic structures of the transition states for various standard reactions could be used as the basis for rapidly building specific transition state structures. For this purpose, substituent groups could be added to calculated reaction centres with the aid of either chemical intuition or classical potential energy calculations.

Identification of Stable Analogues

The major aim of transition state analogue design is to produce a stable molecule which places functional groups in the right positions to bind to corresponding groups in the active site of the enzyme. Because of the long partial bonds of transition state structures this aim can never be achieved precisely. Nevertheless, a reasonable match can often be obtained by designing compounds which mimic the hybridization state of the proposed transition state structure while incorporating one or more atoms with larger covalent radii than those in the substrate. The transition state for the reaction catalysed by cytidine deaminase (Scheme 1), for example, should be matched reasonably accurately by compound (1) (Bartlett *et al.*, 1978). We define this structure as a *topological analogue* of the transition state, since both its atomic connectivity and its hybridization state correspond closely to those of the proposed transition state.

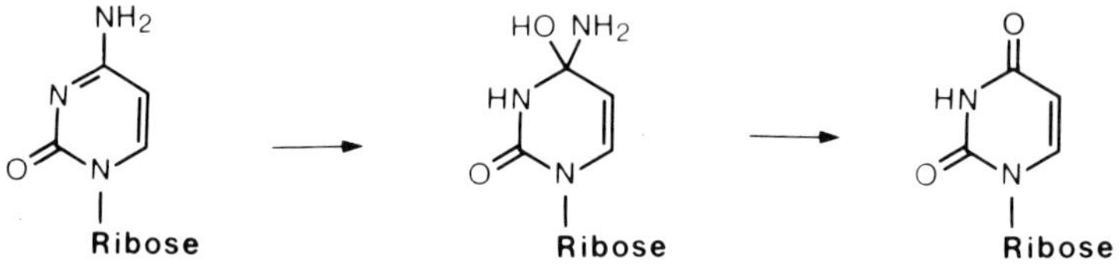

Scheme 1

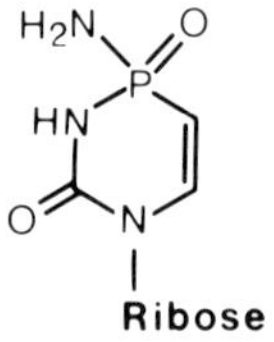

1

In many cases it is not possible to mimic the postulated transition state hybridization so precisely. For the partial reaction shown in Scheme 2, for example, the probable transition state hybridization is intermediate between sp^2 and sp^3, and cannot be precisely analogued. Approximate analogues for this reaction could be (2), in which the methylene substituted for the amide imino protects the labile peptide bond, or (3), in which the phosphinic acid group matches the hybridization state of the metastable reaction intermediate. Neither of these analogues provides a complete topological match to the proposed transition state structure, but both may be sufficiently flexible to allow

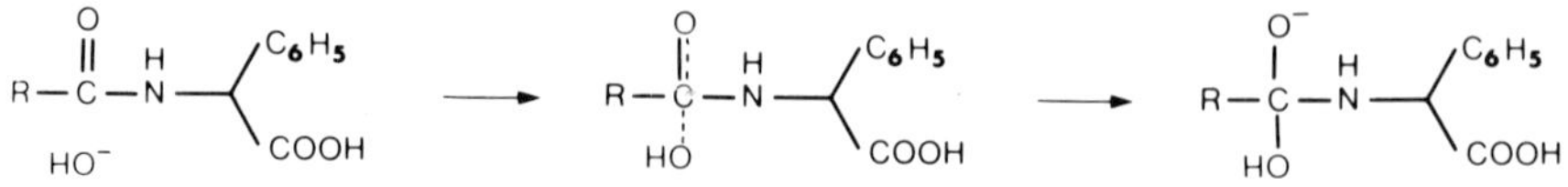

Scheme 2

the appropriate binding groups (R, O, Φ, COOH) to interact with their binding partners in the active site. They may therefore be defined as *topographical* transition state analogues, which match the overall shape of the transition state, and particularly the position and orientation of its binding groups, without precisely matching its topology.

The concept of topographical transition state analogues may be further extended to include structures which bear no obvious relationship to the original reaction mechanism, but simply provide a rigid backbone upon which substituent groups can be correctly orientated to form strong interactions with the enzyme. Compound (4), for example, could be such a topographical analogue for the reaction given in Scheme 2.

Graphs or graphics?
Traditionally the term transition state analogue has been restricted to topological analogues and those topographical analogues which share most of their structural features with a reaction intermediate. This is particularly true of the intuitive approach, which is usually based on the resemblance between *two-dimensional* chemical representations of the transition state and its analogue. With the advent of computer graphic techniques, however, it has become possible to screen large numbers of *three-dimensional* structures as potential analogues for a calculated transition state structure. In our laboratory this is done by superimposing three-dimensional images of the analogues on that of the transition state structure using interactive graphics routines. This process can be automated to allow minimization of the sum of the squares of the distances between corresponding atoms in the two molecules as a function of rotational, translational and conformational variables (Andrews, 1979). Analogues which best fit the proposed transition state structure are then selected for synthesis and testing.

Medicinal Applications of Transition State Analogues

In the following sections we make no attempt to discuss every transition state analogue of medicinal interest, but restrict our attention to four major drug classes where transition state analogues have current or potential therapeutic significance. In most cases these examples also serve to illustrate some specific feature of the transition state analogue approach. Additional examples of medicinal interest are given in the reviews of Lindquist (1975), Wolfenden (1979), Brodbeck (1981) and Ngo and Tunnicliff (1981).

Antihypertensives

Angiotensin converting enzyme (ACE) converts the inactive decapeptide angiotensin I to a potent vasopressor octapeptide, angiotensin II. It also inactivates the powerful vasodepressor, bradykinin. This enzyme is therefore a prime target for antihypertensive drug design.

The recent development of orally active ACE inhibitors was initially based on extensive studies of related peptidases. Of particular importance was the discovery of the powerful carboxypeptidase A inhibitor (R)−benzylsuccinic acid (5), derived from the corresponding substrate (6) by substitution of a methylene group for the imino function of the scissile peptide bond (Byers and Wolfenden, 1973). This compound was

$$HO-\overset{\overset{O}{\|}}{C}-CH_2-\overset{\overset{CH_2C_6H_5}{|}}{CH}-COOH$$

5

$$-\overset{\overset{R}{|}}{CH}-\overset{\overset{O}{\|}}{C}-\overset{H}{N}-C\overset{\diagup R}{\diagdown COOH}$$

6

described by the authors as a biproduct analogue, but examination of the lengths of the peptide bond, or its equivalent, in the substrate, transition state, products and inhibitors of carboxypeptidase A suggests that it is more likely to be a transition state analogue. Table 1 shows that this distance is much greater in the products, where it is determined by the van der Waals' radii, than the apparent optimum separation ($1.5 \text{Å} < x < 2.5 \text{Å}$) suggested by the potencies of the dicarboxylic acid inhibitors. The latter distance is close to that expected in the transition state structure.

By analogy with (5), and bearing in mind the structure−activity relationships of existing peptidic ACE inhibitors from snake venom, Cushman *et al.* (1977) developed the dicarboxylic acid ACE inhibitor, (7), and subsequent structural modification led to the clinically useful antihypertensive agent, captopril (8). Like (5), captopril cannot be regarded as a topological transition state analogue, but similar arguments

TABLE 1

Benzylsuccinic acid: biproduct analogue or transition state analogue?

REACTANT OR INHIBITOR	STRUCTURE	PEPTIDE BOND (OR EQUIVALENT) LENGTH Å	K_I (μM)
SUBSTRATE		1.4	
TRANSITION STATE		~1.8	
PRODUCTS		3.2	
BENZYLMALONIC ACID		~0	60
D,L-BENZYLSUCCINIC ACID		1.5	1.1
D,L-BENZYLGLUTARIC ACID		2.5	5

$$HO-\overset{\overset{O}{\|}}{C}-CH_2-CH_2-\overset{\overset{O}{\|}}{C}-N\diagdown_{COOH}$$

$$HS-CH_2-\overset{\overset{CH_3}{|}}{CH}-\overset{\overset{O}{\|}}{C}-N\diagdown_{COOH}$$

7   8

to those above suggest that it may be topographically analogous to the transition state. Support for this view is derived from a comparison between captopril and its major competitor, enalapril (9), for which it is claimed that a transition state-like geometry is attained in the scissile bond region via the $CHCO_2R$ and NH groups (Patchett *et al.*, 1980).

$$C_2H_5-O-\overset{\overset{O}{\|}}{C}-\underset{\underset{\underset{CH_2C_6H_5}{|}}{CH_2}}{\overset{|}{CH}}-\overset{H}{N}-\overset{\overset{CH_3}{|}}{CH}-\overset{\overset{O}{\|}}{C}-N\diagdown_{COOH}$$

9

Stereoscopic views of the lowest energy conformations (A.S. Caselli, R.A. Woods, J.M. Carson, P.R. Andrews, unpublished results) of captopril and the diacid metabolite of enalapril are shown in Fig. 1, in which three of the major active site binding groups are positioned to maximize their interactions with the corresponding functional groups of the inhibitors. Despite the topological differences between these two inhibitors, it is clear that their stereochemical interactions with the active site are very similar indeed.

Many other potent ACE inhibitors have been developed over the past few years, and their structure–activity relationships have recently been reviewed (Petrillo and Ondetti, 1982). These include compounds designed to approximate the geometry of the transition state, such as (10) (Thorsett *et al.*, 1982) and others whose potencies rely more on topographical similarities, e.g. (11) (Meyer *et al.*, 1981). These data thus provide an opportunity to determine the relative importance of topological and topographical analogies to the transition state structure.

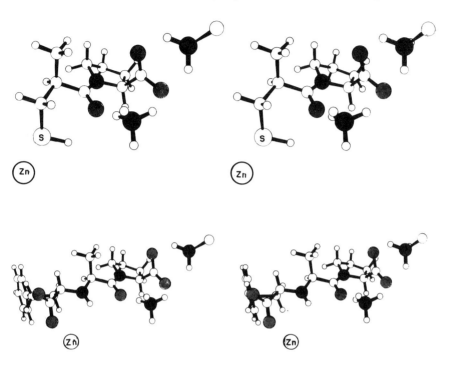

FIG. 1 Stereoscopic views* of captopril (8, top) and the diacid metabolite of enalapril (9, bottom) in a three-dimensional model binding site comprising Zn^{++} and two basic groups capable of forming a hydrogen bond to the carbonyl oxygen and an ionic bond to the carboxyl terminal. Light and dark shadings represent oxygen and nitrogen, respectively.

10

11

* A "stereo-viewer", suitable for use with Fig. 1 has been designed by Professor F. Vögtle and distributed by Verlag Chemie (obtainable from the Royal Society of Chemistry in England).

Topology or Topography?
The structures collected in Table 2 differ only in their zinc-binding functions, and it is clear that their inhibitory potency depends much more
on the affinity of these functional groups for zinc than on their
topological resemblance to the (presumably) tetrahedral transition state
structure. Topology for its own sake thus appears to be unimportant,
although in some cases the correct topology may have the desirable

TABLE 2

Effect of varying zinc-binding function on inhibitor potency (Petrillo and Ondetti, 1982)

$$X-CH_2-CH_2-\overset{\overset{\textstyle O}{\|}}{C}-N\overset{}{\underset{COOH}{\diagdown}}$$

X	I_{50} (μM)
$HO-\overset{\overset{\textstyle O}{\|}}{\underset{\underset{\textstyle O}{\|}}{S}}-$	> 10,000
$HO-\overset{\overset{\textstyle O}{\|}}{\underset{\underset{\textstyle OH}{\|}}{P}}-$	48
$HO-\overset{\overset{\textstyle O}{\|}}{C}-$	330
$HO-\underset{\underset{\textstyle H}{\|}}{N}-\overset{\overset{\textstyle O}{\|}}{C}-$	0.61
$H-S-$	0.20

consequence of forcing the required positioning of additional distant binding groups (e.g. compound (10), $I_{50} = 0.007 \mu M$, Thorsett *et al.*, 1982). That this may be achieved without the topological constraint is evident in inhibitors such as (11) ($I_{50} = 0.003 \mu M$, Meyer *et al.*, 1981). A further reason for abandoning precise topological analogies is the possibility of developing rigid topographical transition state analogues which may possess a substantial entropic advantage in their binding to the active site of the enzyme. This goal has been partly achieved in the bicyclic ACE inhibitor (12) under development by Hoffmann–La Roche (Hassall and Moody, 1981). It is hoped that the specificity for both substrate and reaction inherent in such rigid transition state analogues will lead to inhibitors devoid of the side-effects which limit the clinical utility of current ACE inhibitors.

$$HS-CH_2-CH_2-N$$

12

Antibacterials

β-lactam antibiotics   The final step in bacterial cell wall synthesis involves the crosslinking of peptidoglycan chains. This process is regulated by various transpeptidases and carboxypeptidases, which catalyse the cleavage of the terminal D–alanyl–D–alanine bond of the glycopeptides. These enzymes are thus suitable targets for antibacterial action, and are among the likely sites of action for the β-lactam antibiotics (Yocum *et al.*, 1979).

It was suggested by Tipper and Strominger (1965) and by Lee (1971) that the nonplanar amide bond of the penicillins (13), could resemble a possible transition state structure for the cleavage of the D–alanyl–D–alanine peptide bond. This possibility has been tested by Boyd (1977), who used MINDO/3 to calculate reaction pathways for the nucleophilic attack of a hydroxyl ion from above (β) or below (α) the carbonyl carbon of a model dipeptide, glycylglycine (14). No high energy barrier, and therefore no transition state structure, was located on either pathway in the gas phase, but the calculations identified stable tetrahedral transition intermediates for attack on either face. These

O
‖   H
R—C—N
                S
                    CH₃
            N   CH₃
O
        COOH

O
‖   H
NH₂—CH₂ —C —N —CH₂COOH

13   14

structures, which could be intermediates or transition states on a condensed-phase reaction surface, were too close in energy to discriminate between the alternative reaction pathways.

Conformational calculations on the substrate and on the alternative transition intermediates showed that all three structures are sufficiently flexible to provide a reasonable topographical match to a range of β-lactam antibiotics (Boyd, 1979). Figure 2 illustrates the structural analogy between a model β-lactam structure, 6-amino-3-carboxylpenam, derived from the crystal structure of potassium penicillin G (Dexter and van der Veen, 1978), and the corresponding calculated conformations of glycylglycine and the slightly preferred α-face transition intermediate (Boyd, 1977, 1979). On the basis of these data, the β-lactam antibiotics may be regarded as either substrate or transition state analogues for the bacterial cell wall peptidases.

Regardless of their initial binding, many of the β-lactams subsequently acylate functional groups in the active site of the peptidases, and the extent of their activity can be correlated with the calculated reactivity of the β-lactam ring (Boyd and Lunn, 1979). The β-lactam antibiotics may thus combine, to some degree, the virtues of both transition state analogues and mechanism-based irreversible inhibitors.

Shikimate pathway   The shikimate pathway is a vital source of aromatic amino acids in bacteria and plants, but is absent in man (Haslam, 1974). It is thus a potential, but as yet underutilized, target for antibacterial drugs.

Molecular orbital calculations have been carried out on two of the reactions in the shikimate pathway (Schemes 3 and 4). Both of these reactions are catalysed by the same bifunctional enzyme in several bacterial species (Andrews and Heyde, 1979). For the Claisen rearrangement of chorismate to prephenate (Scheme 3), the calculations located two alternative transition states (Andrews *et al.*, 1973; Andrews and Haddon, 1979). These result from the clockwise and anticlockwise

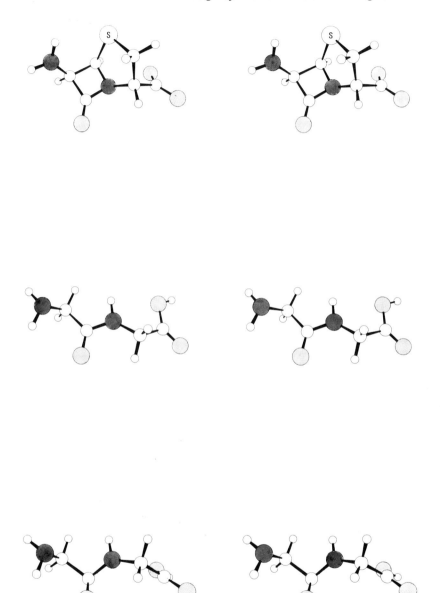

FIG. 2   Stereoscopic views of a model β-lactam structure (top) and calculated conformations of glycylglycine (middle) and the α-face transition intermediate (bottom). Attack by the hydroxyl ion (not shown) is on the far side of the carbonyl carbon. The three structures are orientated to illustrate the similarities in position and orientation of the amine, carbonyl and carboxyl groups thought to be involved in binding to the active site (Boyd, 1979). Light and dark shadings represent oxygen and nitrogen, respectively.

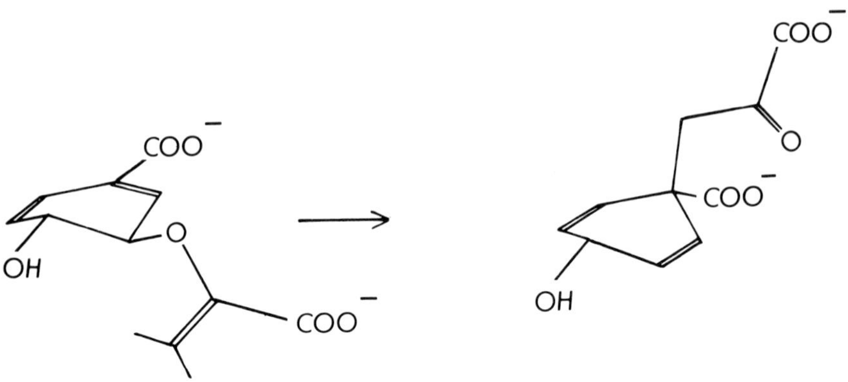

Scheme 3

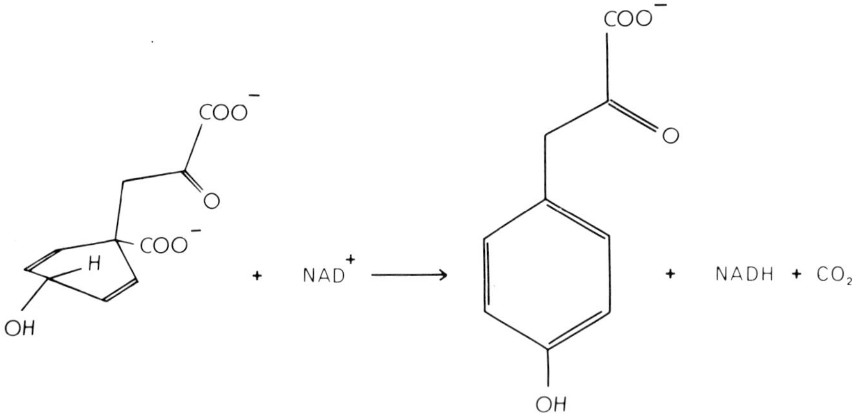

Scheme 4

rotation of the side chain around the breaking C–O bond, and adopt chair-like and boat-like conformations respectively (Fig. 3). The calculated energy difference between the two alternatives is too small to define a preferred transition state structure. Analogues of both transition states were therefore synthesized and tested in the expectation that the analogue resembling the true transition state would be identified by the strength of the observed inhibition. This proved to be the case, with the chair-like analogue (Fig. 3c) being the much more potent inhibitor (Andrews *et al.*, 1977). Similar inhibition is seen in the adamantane derivative (Fig. 3e), in which the chair conformation is fixed by the addition of a methylene group. The inhibition data thus indicate that the transition state for the enzyme catalysed reaction is the chair-like intermediate. This example illustrates an advantage of calculating

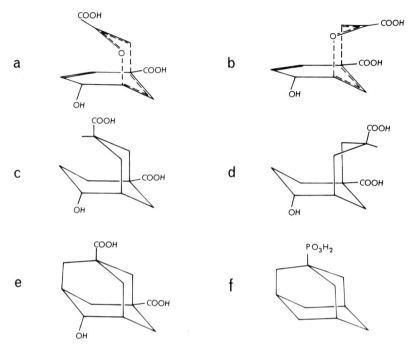

FIG. 3 Diagrammatic representations of the alternative transition state structures, and some proposed analogues, for the isomerisation of chorismate to prephenate: (a) chair-like transition state structure; (b) boat-like transition state structure; (c) chair-like nonane analogue; (d) boat-like nonane analogue; (e) chair-like adamantane analogue; (f) adamantane-1-phosphonic acid.

complete reaction surfaces, namely, that all likely transition states are identified at the outset, and inhibition by analogues can then be used to specify the correct transition state structure (Andrews, 1979).

Thermodynamic measurements on the same enzyme show a substantial decrease in the entropy of activation for the enzyme catalysed isomerization (Görisch, 1978) relative to the nonenzymatic reaction (Andrews *et al.*, 1973), which suggests that the topographical requirements of the active site are rather tight (Görisch, 1978). This view is confirmed by structure–activity studies on the adamantane inhibitors, which show that the second carboxyl group is not properly aligned to interact with the receptor (Andrews, 1979). The strength of the inhibition due to adamantane-1-carboxylic acid (Andrews *et al.*, 1977) and the corresponding phosphonate (Fig. 3f), which is the most powerful known inhibitor of the enzyme (Chao and Berchtold, 1982), indicates that the adamantanes are primarily topographical analogues whose hydrocarbon skeleton plays a major role in binding to the enzyme. This example thus illustrates the importance of topographical analogy in the design of transition state inhibitors.

The latter point is further emphasized by calculations on the second reaction (Scheme 4). If, as is thought, both reactions are catalysed at the same active site, we would expect very similar transition states for the two reactions. Comparison of the two transition states interacting with a proposed active site model (Fig. 4), shows that while the topological resemblance between the two structures is slight, the placement and orientation of the important binding groups are virtually identical (Andrews and Heyde, 1979).

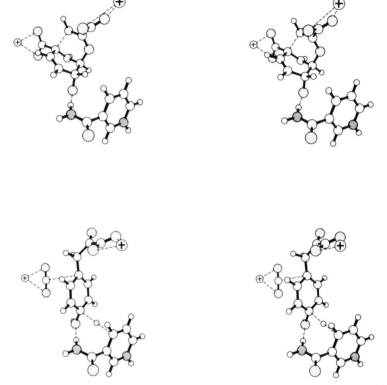

FIG. 4   Stereoscopic comparison of the transition states for the isomerisation of chorismate (top) and the dehydrogenation of prephenate (bottom) in a three-dimensional model of the active site. The model consists of the nicotinamide ring of NAD and two positively charged groups capable of forming ionic bonds to the carboxyl groups of the transition states. Light and dark shadings represent oxygen and nitrogen, respectively.

Nature or science?

Although the adamantane inhibitors (Fig. 3) are a clear result of computer-assisted drug design, the β-lactam antibiotics are equally clearly derived from natural origins. How does nature compare with science in the design of other antibacterial transition state analogues?

The antibiotic coformycin (15) is one of a number of apparent transition state analogues isolated from natural sources (Umezawa, 1972). It resembles the probable tetrahedral intermediate (16) for the adenosine deaminase catalysed attack of water on adenosine, binding approximately one million times more tightly than the substrate (Cha *et al.*, 1975).

15   16

The related compounds 2'-deoxycoformycin (Woo *et al.*, 1974) and 2'-deoxycoformycin-5'-phosphate (Frieden *et al.*, 1979) are equally potent inhibitors of adenosine deaminase and AMP deaminase, respectively. In each of these compounds there is a clear topological analogy to the tetrahedral group in the proposed transition state, but the extra methylene group in the analogues must perform some topographical function in determining the precise location of the additional binding groups. The position of the ribose substituent in particular appears to be very important (Wolfenden, 1978). It will be interesting to compare the activities of these natural antibiotics with those of the purely topological analogues (17) being developed by Bartlett *et al.*, 1978).

The design provided by nature in coformycin has also been adapted, with some success, in the development of related inhibitors (18) for bacterial cytidine deaminase (Marquez *et al.*, 1980). These are

17

18   19

approximately ten times more powerful than the already potent topological analogue, 3,4,5,6-tetrahydrouridine (19) (Camiener, 1968).

Another of the natural transition state analogues is the antibiotic
nojirimycin, of which the dehydrated form (20) is a clear topological
analogue of the postulated cationic intermediate (21) for glucosidase
hydrolysis (Reese *et al.*, 1971). A similar principle has been applied by
Flashner *et al.* (1979) in the design of neuraminidase inhibitors.

20   21

Anticonvulsants

A potential target for anticonvulsant drug action is GABA-transaminase, which is responsible for the destruction of the inhibitory neurotransmitter, γ-aminobutyric acid (GABA), in the mammalian central
nervous system. This potential is confirmed by the anticonvulsant
activity of several mechanism-based irreversible inhibitors of GABA-
transaminase developed by Metcalf (1979). Multisubstrate analogues
of GABA-transaminase have also been developed with varying degrees
of success (Severin *et al.*, 1969; Tunnicliff *et al.*, 1977).

Molecular orbital calculations have been used to calculate the
potential energy surface for the rate determining tautomeric step in the
reaction catalysed by GABA-transaminase (Scheme 5). Studies on model
reactions and various transaminases suggest that this reaction is base
catalysed, probably by a lysine residue, and proceeds in a *cis* manner
(Walsh, 1979). The initial calculations were therefore carried out on

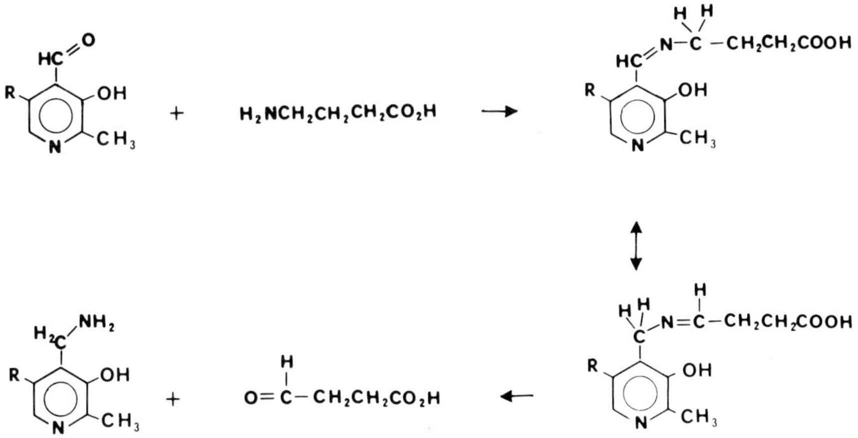

Scheme 5

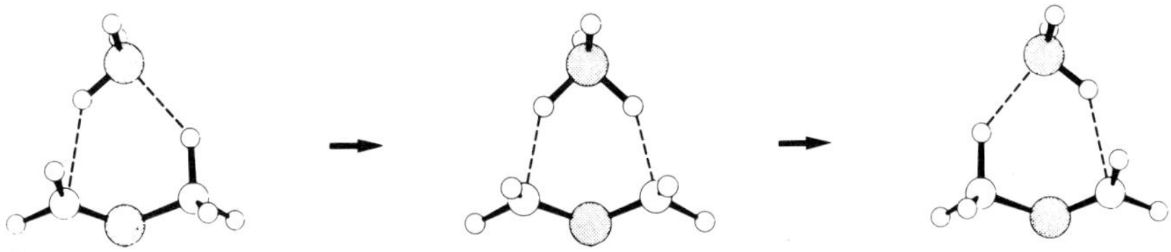

FIG. 5   Model reaction representing the tautomeric step in GABA-transamination. The shaded atoms are nitrogens and the group at the top is the onium head of the lysine thought to be involved as the catalytic base.

the simple model reaction shown in Fig. 5. Despite the two hydrogen transfers involved, both MINDO/3 (Andrews *et al.*, 1982) and MNDO (D.A. Winkler and P.R. Andrews, unpublished results) gave a smooth transition from reactants to products, although a thorough analysis of the reaction surface probably requires a multiconfigurational *ab initio* treatment (Maggiora and Christoffersen, 1978).

The calculated transition state structure is a symmetric ion pair with N–H bonds of ~1.2 Å and C–H bonds ~1.5 Å. Subsequent incorporation of the 3-hydroxypyridine group led to a planar transition state structure stabilized by a hydrogen bond from the 3-hydroxyl moiety. The conformations of the remaining substituents were then optimized using classical potential energy calculations to give the final structure illustrated in Fig. 6 (Andrews *et al.*, 1982).

The planarity of the calculated transition state structure suggests that cyclic derivatives of GABA with pyridoxal phosphate would be suitable transition state analogues, and computer graphic comparisons showed

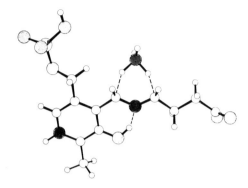

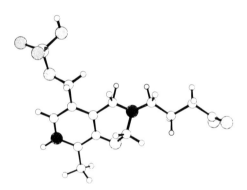

FIG. 6   Structural comparison of the calculated transition state (top) and a proposed pyridoxazine transition state analogue (bottom) for the reaction catalysed by GABA-transaminase. The onium head of the lysine thought to be involved in the hydrogen transfer is included in the transition state structure. Light and dark shadings represent oxygen and nitrogen, respectively.

that a good match to the transition state structure could be obtained with the corresponding pyridoxazine (Fig. 6).

Synthesis and preliminary testing of several molecules in this series gave mixed results (M.N. Iskander, P. Beart, G.P. Jones, P. Mclennan, D.A. Winkler and P.R. Andrews, unpublished results). Inhibition of GABA-transaminase *in vitro* required millimolar concentrations of inhibitor, while anticonvulsant activity *in vivo* appeared to develop slowly over a period of days. These observations, although tentative, suggest that the activity of these inhibitors may be determined less by their potency than by the tenacity with which the coenzyme retains its grip on the active site.

Reversible or irreversible?
While the preceding efforts to design transition state analogues of GABA-transaminase have so far met with limited success, the design of irreversible mechanism-based inhibitors for the same enzyme has led to inhibitors with clinical potential as anticonvulsants (Metcalf, 1979). Are transition state analogues a worthwhile alternative?

The major advantages of irreversible inhibition are the very high potency conferred by the formation of a covalent bond to the active site, and the relative simplicity of designing and synthesizing inhibitors that are essentially substrate analogues. The major disadvantages arise from the same factors: enzyme specificity is determined only at the substrate level, and activity may not be reversible even when this is therapeutically desirable.

Transition state analogues owe their equally high potency to the sum total of many noncovalent bonds specified by the structural complementarity of the transition state structure and the active site. Specificity for the target enzyme should therefore be extremely high, although the effort required to design and synthesize transition state analogues will be correspondingly increased.

In many respects the two approaches are complementary, and both appear well worth pursuing. It may also prove possible to combine some of their merits in the design of irreversible transition state analogues. As noted above, the β-lactam antibiotics may be naturally occurring examples of this class.

Antineoplastic Agents

The enzymes of the *de novo* pyrimidine pathway are potential targets for new antineoplastic drugs (Kensler and Cooney, 1981). Transition state analogues have been developed for two sites in the pathway.

Collins and Stark (1971) designed the aspartate transcarbamylase inhibitor N-(phosphonoacetyl)-L-aspartate (PALA), (22)) on the basis of its analogy to the postulated transition state structure, (23). Both PALA and the corresponding methylene derivative (24) are extremely potent inhibitors, having K_i values of the same order as the product of the substrate dissociation constants (Swyryd *et al.*, 1974). These and related inhibitors (Goodson *et al.*, 1980) are all sp^2 hybridized at the reaction centre, and are therefore topographical analogues of the postulated tetrahedral reaction intermediate.

1-(5'-Phospho-β-D-ribofuranosyl) barbituric acid (25) inhibits orotidine-5'-phosphate decarboxylase with a K_i of 9×10^{-12} M, the tightest known binding between an enzyme and a synthetic inhibitor (Levine *et al.*, 1980). The inhibitor is anionic at physiological pH but

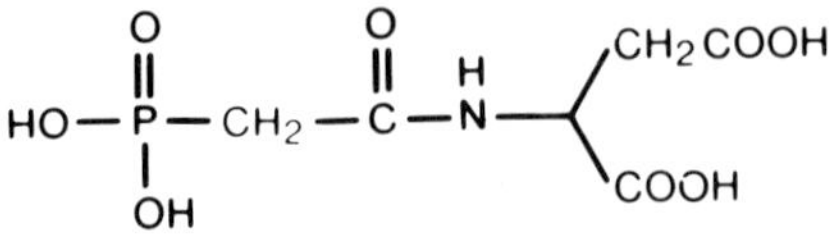

22

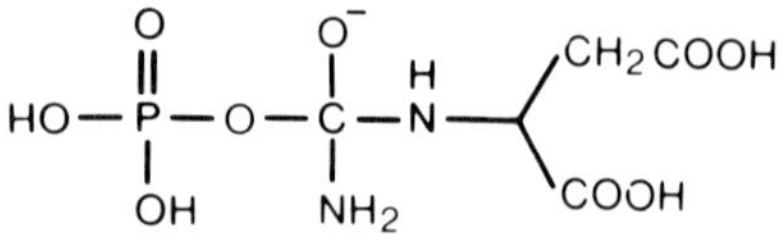

23

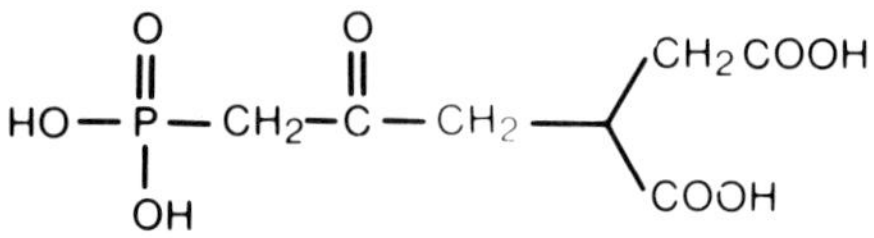

24

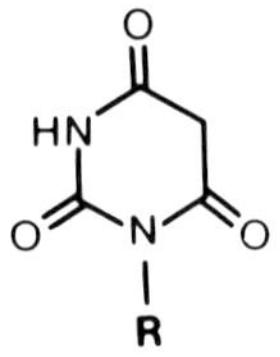

25

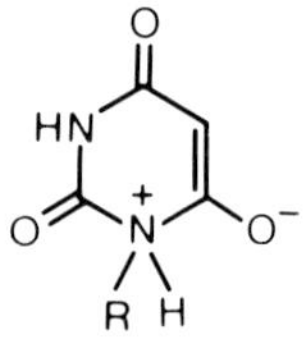

26

may be protonated in the active site to yield the zwitterion, (26). The latter structure is topographically intermediate between the zwitterionic and nitrogen ylide transition states on the postulated reaction pathway (Scheme 6, Beak and Siegel, 1976).

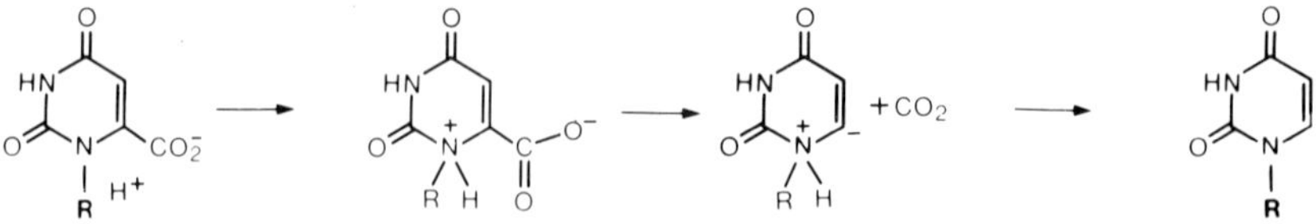

Scheme 6

Accident or design?
The preceding two examples also serve to illustrate some of the uncertainties still inherent in the drug design process. In the case of the barbiturate (25), for example, the role of transition state analogue was advanced (Levine *et al.*, 1980) as an explanation for its extraordinary potency rather than as the basis for its development (Potvin *et al.*, 1978). The successful design of PALA, on the other hand, makes its postulated role as a transition state analogue extremely attractive, but Heyde (1976) has suggested that this is not the most likely interpretation of the kinetic and spectral data. She proposes that PALA binds at the carbamyl phosphate subsite and an adjacent anionic binding site, leaving the binding site for the second substrate, aspartate, unoccupied. Serendipity may thus still prove responsible for this successful example of drug design.

On the credit side for drug design are the increased availability of structural and mechanistic data for many target enzymes, and major recent advances in computational and computer graphic techniques. Thus, for example, the superficially surprising suggestion that dihydrofolate may bind to dihydrofolate reductase upside down with respect to its topological "analogue" methotrexate (Charlton *et al.*, 1979) turns out to be entirely predictable on the basis of conformational energy and electrostatic potential calculations of the two structures (Spark *et al.*, 1982).

Conclusion

As shown in the preceding survey, it is not too difficult to find examples of transition state analogues with medicinal applications, and there are also a number of examples of successful transition state analogue design. It is not so easy, however, to identify examples of transition state analogues which combine successful design and therapeutic utility. PALA (22) and the angiotensin converting enzyme inhibitors captopril (8) and enalapril (9) are perhaps the outstanding examples, although captopril was not intended as a transition state analogue.

Each of these inhibitors is a topographical, rather than topological, analogue of the corresponding transition state structure. This suggests that the primary considerations in the design of new transition state analogues should be the correct position and orientation of the substituent binding groups. In these examples, the conformational flexibility of the inhibitors may also contribute significantly to their ability to bind at the active site, but more potent analogues could conceivably be designed by incorporating the "correct" placement of the binding groups in a rigid analogue of the transition state structure. The natural antibiotic coformycin (15) and the barbiturate (25) are examples of highly potent semirigid transition state analogues.

The future development of entirely rigid analogues will be substantially aided by the use of computer graphic techniques to match calculated transition state structures. These techniques should be particularly helpful in predicting novel inhibitor structures such as the adamantanes (Fig. 3), which bear little obvious resemblance to the reactants in the inhibited reaction (Scheme 3).

Fact or fantasy?

As noted at the outset, the choice of examples for this survey was restricted to those with clear medicinal applications. Implicit in this restriction is the eventual criterion for the success or failure of the method – "Can it provide new drugs?". If this were the only criterion then the transition state analogue approach to drug design would undoubtedly be "fantasy", since it takes no account of the metabolic or other pharmacokinetic requirements for drug action. Indeed, the sole purpose of the transition state analogue approach is the design of novel and potent enzyme inhibitors, for which a more appropriate criterion is – "Can it provide new leads?". On this basis, the undoubted success of these techniques in the design of novel enzyme inhibitors (Wolfenden, 1976) unequivocally labels the transition state analogue approach as "fact". Other techniques, many of which are discussed in this volume, must then be used to convert the leads generated by the transition state analogue approach into new drugs.

Acknowledgements

We are grateful to Jim Burchall, Gerry Maggiora, Garland Marshall, Yvonne Martin and Richard Wolfenden for their valuable comments, and to Cathy Balderstone for typing the manuscript.

References

Albert, A. (1979). "Selective Toxicity". Chapman and Hall, London.
Andrews, P.R. (1979). *In* "Computer-Assisted Drug Design" (E.C. Olson and R.E. Christoffersen, eds.), American Chemical Society Symposium Series **112**, 149–159.
Andrews, P.R., Cain, E.N., Rizzardo, E. and Smith, G.D. (1977). *Biochemistry* **16**, 4848–4852.
Andrews, P.R. and Haddon, R.C. (1979). *Aust. J. Chem.* **32**, 1921–1929.
Andrews, P.R. and Heyde, E. (1979). *J. Theor. Biol.* **78**, 393–403.
Andrews, P.R., Iskander, M.N., Jones, G.P. and Winkler, D.A. (1982). *Int. J. Quantum Chem.: Quantum Biol. Symp.* **9**, 345–353.
Andrews, P.R., Smith, G.D. and Young, I.G. (1973). *Biochemistry* **12**, 3492–3498.

Baker, B.R. (1967). "Design of Active-Site-Directed Irreversible Enzyme Inhibitors. The Organic Chemistry of the Enzymic Active-Site." Wiley, New York.

Bartlett, P.A., Hunt, J.T., Adams, J.L. and Gehret, J.-C.E. (1978). *Bioorg. Chem.* 7, 421–436.

Beak, P. and Siegel, B. (1976). *J. Am. Chem. Soc.* 98, 3601–3606.

Bernstein F.C., Koetzle, T.F., Williams, G.J.B., Meyer, E.F., Brice, M.D. *et al.* (1977). *J. Mol. Biol.* 112, 535–542.

Bingham, R.C., Dewar, M.J.S. and Lo, D.H. (1975). *J. Am. Chem. Soc.* 97, 1285–1293.

Boyd, D.B. (1977). *Proc. Natl. Acad. Sci. U.S.A.* 74, 5239–5243.

Boyd, D.B. (1979). *J. Med. Chem.* 22, 533–537.

Boyd, D.B. and Lunn, W.H.W. (1979). *J. Antibiot.* 32, 855–856.

Brodbeck, U. (1981). *In* "Enzyme Inhibitors" (U. Brodbeck, ed.), pp. 3–17. Verlag Chemie, Weinheim.

Byers, L.D. and Wolfenden, R. (1973). *Biochemistry* 12, 2070–2078.

Camiener, G.W. (1968). *Biochem. Pharmacol.* 17, 1981–1991.

Cha, S., Agarwal, R.P. and Parks, R.E. (1975). *Biochem. Pharmacol.* 24, 2187–2197.

Chao, H.S.I. and Berchtold, G.A. (1982). Private communication.

Charlton, P.A., Young, D.W., Birdsall, B., Feeney, J. and Roberts, G.C.K. (1979). *J. Chem. Soc. Chem. Commun.*, 922–924.

Collins, K.D. and Stark, G.R. (1971). *J. Biol. Chem.* 246, 6599–6605.

Cushman, D.W., Cheung, H.S., Sabo, E.F. and Ondetti, M.A. (1977). *Biochemistry* 16, 5484–5491.

Dedieu, A. and Veillard, A. (1970). *Chem. Phys. Lett.* 5, 328–330.

Dewar, M.J.S. and Kirschner, S. (1971a). *J. Am. Chem. Soc.* 93, 4291–4292.

Dewar, M.J.S. and Kirschner, S. (1971b). *J. Am. Chem. Soc.* 93, 4292–4294.

Dewar, M.J.S. and Kirschner, S. (1974). *J. Am. Chem. Soc.* 96, 5244–5246.

Dewar, M.J.S. and Thiel, W. (1977). *J. Am. Chem. Soc.* 99, 4899–4907.

Dexter, D.D. and van der Veen, J.M. (1978). *J. Chem. Soc. Perkin Trans. I*, 185–190.

Flashner, M., Kessler, J. and Tanenbaum, S.W. (1979). *In* "Drug Action and Design: Mechanism-based Enzyme Inhibitors" (T.I. Kalman, ed.), pp. 27–44, Elsevier North Holland, New York.

Frieden, C., Gilbert, H.R., Miller, W.H. and Miller, R.I. (1979) *Biochem. Biophys. Res. Commun.* 91, 278–283.

Gandour, R.D. and Schowen, R.L., eds (1978). "Transition States of Biochemical Processes". Plenum Press, New York.

Goodson, J.J., Wharton, C.J. and Wrigglesworth, R. (1980). *J. Chem. Soc. Perkin Trans. I*, 2721–2727.

Görisch, H. (1978). *Biochemistry* 17, 3700–3705.

Halgren, T.A. and Lipscomb, W.N. (1973). *J. Chem. Phys.* 58, 1569–1591.

Haslam, E. (1974). "The Shikimate Pathway". Butterworths, London.

Hassall, C.H. and Moody, C.J. (1981). Triazolpyridazinderivative, Verfahren und Zwischenprodukte zu ihrer Herstellung, diese enthaltende Arzneimittel und deren therapeutische Verwendung. European Patent 0 024 309 A2.

Heyde, E. (1976). *Biochim. Biophys. Acta* 452, 81–88.

Jug, K. (1980). *Theor. Chim. Acta* 54, 263–300.

Kensler, T.W. and Cooney, D.A. (1981). *In* "Advances in Pharmacology and Chemotherapy", Vol. 18 (S. Garottini, A. Goldin, F. Hawking and I.J. Kopin, eds), pp. 273–352. Academic Press, New York.

Lee, B. (1971). *J. Mol. Biol.* 61, 463–469.

Levine, H.L., Brody, R.S. and Westheimer, F.H. (1980). *Biochemistry* 19, 4993–4999.

Lienhard, G.E. (1972). *Annu. Rep. Med. Chem.* **7**, 249–258.
Lienhard, G.E. (1973). *Science* **180**, 149–154.
Lindquist, R.N. (1975). *In* "Drug Design", Vol. 5 (E.J. Ariëns, ed.), 23–80. Academic Press, New York.
Maggiora, G.M. and Christoffersen, R.E. (1978). *In* "Transition States of Biochemical Processes". (R.D. Gandour and R.L. Schowen, eds), 119–163, Plenum Press, New York.
Marquez, V.E., Liu, P.S., Kelley, J.A., Driscoll, J.S. and McCormack, J.J. (1980). *J. Med. Chem.* **23**, 713–715.
Matthews, D.A., Alden, R.A., Bolin, J.T., Filman, D.J., Freer, S.T. *et al.* (1978). *J. Biol. Chem.* **253**, 6946–6954.
McIver, J.W. and Komornicki, A. (1972). *J. Am. Chem. Soc.* **94**, 2625–2633.
Metcalf, B.W. (1979). *Biochem. Pharmacol.* **28**, 1705–1712.
Meyer, R.F., Nicolaides, E.D., Tinney, F.J., Lunney, E.A., Holmes, A. *et al.* (1981). *J. Med. Chem.* **24**, 964–969.
Murrell, J.N. and Laidler, K.J. (1968). *Trans. Faraday Soc.* **64**, 371–377.
Ngo, T.T. and Tunnicliff, G. (1981). *Gen. Pharmacol.* **12**, 129–138.
Patchett, A.A., Harris, E., Tristram, E.W., Wyvratt, M.J., Wu, M.T. *et al.* (1980). *Nature* (London) **288**, 280–283.
Pauling, L. (1946). *Chem. Eng. News* **24**, 1375–1377.
Petrillo, E.W. and Ondetti, M.A. (1982). *Med. Res. Rev.* **2**, 1–41.
Potvin, B.W., Stern, H.J., May, S.R., Lam, G.F. and Krooth, R.S. (1978). *Biochem. Pharmacol.* **27**, 655–665.
Rando, R.R. (1974). *Science* **185**, 320–324.
Reese, E.T., Parrish, F.W. and Ettlinger, M. (1971). *Carbohydr. Res.* **18**, 381–388.
Scheiner, S. (1980). *Theor. Chim. Acta* **57**, 71–80.
Schlegel, H.B. (1982). *J. Comput. Chem.* **3**, 214–218.
Severin, E.S., Gulyaev, N.N., Khurs, E.N. and Khomutov, R.M. (1969). *Biochem. Biophys. Res. Commun.* **35**, 318–323.
Spark, M.J., Winkler, D.A. and Andrews, P.R. (1982). *Int. J. Quantum Chem.: Quantum Biol. Symp.* **9**, 321–333.
Spangler, D., Williams, I.H. and Maggiora, G.M. (1982). Private communication.
Swyryd, E.A., Seaver, S.A. and Stark, G.A. (1974). *J. Biol. Chem.* **249**, 6945–6950.
Thorsett, E.D., Harris, E.E., Peterson, E.R., Greenlee, W.J., Patchett, A.A., Ulm, E.H. and Vassil, T.C. (1982). *Proc. Natl. Acad. Sci. U.S.A.* **79**, 2176–2180.
Tipper, D.J. and Strominger, J.L. (1965). *Proc. Natl. Acad. Sci. U.S.A.* **54**, 1133–1141.
Tunnicliff, G., Ngo, T.T. and Barbeau, A. (1977). *Experientia* **33**, 20–22.
Umezawa, H. (1972). "Enzyme Inhibitors of Microbial Origin". University Park Press, Baltimore.
Walsh, C. (1979). "Enzymatic Reaction Mechanism". Freeman and Company, San Francisco.
Wolfenden, R. (1969). Transition state analogues for enzyme catalysis. *Nature* (London) **223**, 704–705.
Wolfenden, R. (1972). *Acc. Chem. Res.* **5**, 10–18.
Wolfenden, R. (1976). *Annu. Rev. Biophys. Bioeng.* **5**, 271–306.
Wolfenden, R. (1978). *In* "Transition States of Biochemical Processes" (R.D. Gandour and R.L. Schowen, eds), pp. 555–578. Plenum Press, New York.
Wolfenden, R. (1979). *In* "Antimetabolites in Biochemistry, Biology and Medicine" (J. Skoda and P. Langen, eds), pp. 151–160. Pergamon, Oxford.
Woo, P.K., Dion, H.W., Lange, S.M., Dahl, L.F. and Durham, L.J. (1974). *J. Heterocycl. Chem.* **11**, 641–643.

Yocum, R.R., Waxman, D.J., Rasmussen, J.R. and Strominger, J.L. (1979). *Proc. Natl. Acad. Sci. U.S.A.* **76**, 2730–2734.

Discussion

Chairman: Professor Tomlinson

Dr Dearden
Professor Andrews has shown how these transition state analogues must certainly be extremely precise in the way they fit the receptor. But, of course, they also have to get to the receptor. Is there any evidence that there is a need to build in a certain level of lipophilicity, for example, to enable the compound to get to the receptor site, or is the fact that it mimics a natural substrate generally sufficient to get it to the appropriate receptor site?

Professor Andrews
It certainly cannot be assumed that because a transition state analogue mimics a natural substrate it will necessarily get to the site of action. Frequently, the natural substrate is already at the site, having been formed there. I would really like to pass the buck back to the QSAR and pro-drug people, and say that it is their job to optimize the lead compounds developed by the transition state analogue approach in order to ensure that they reach the site of action.

There are, however, some cases where a transition state analogue may never be able to reach the site of action. For example, if a transition state analogue was made for dihydrofolate reductase as a combination of dihydrofolate and NADPH, it would never properly occupy the active site because the two subsites are separated by a narrow channel (which can be seen in the crystal structure) through which neither of the individual substrates could pass, although it provides the environment for hydrogen transfer from one to the other.

Dr Bowden
Is there any real distinction that can possibly be made between the transition state analogue and the product, or the real substrate analogue, in such a system? By definition, the reaction co-ordinate between the initial state and the product lies through the transition state, and there is really a continuum. Is there any real guideline by which it would be possible to say that one was a real transition state analogue, as opposed to a substrate or product analogue?

Professor Andrews
It is certainly difficult. People have tended to go on the potency of the compound — saying that if it is extremely potent, then it is a transition state analogue. That, clearly, is not a precise way of making that definition.

I suppose that the major difference between the transition state, the substrate and the product, as Dr Bowden stated, is the particular positions and orientations of their functional groups as we go through the reaction. It is the match of any particular analogue to what is believed to be the substrate, transition state or product that is the most likely way of making the definition. In many cases, it is a semantic problem. In the case of the penicillin-type compounds, as I have shown today, we really cannot tell.

Dr Bowden
May I reinforce the point that you made. The medicinal chemist using such guidelines would arrive at similar drug systems. The important point after all is not the precise mode of action, but arriving at novel and effective drugs.

Professor Roques
With regard to the compounds made by Merck, the angiotensin-converting enzyme inhibitor, the increasing affinity and potency were attributed by Merck to a more precise similarity to the transition state. As is known, however, there is another reason. There is an addition of a benzyl group in that compound, and it is well-known (for about 10 years now) that there is an additional subsite on the angiotensin coverting enzyme which interacts strongly with a benzyl or other aromatic group. For instance, the replacement of the benzyl group with a methyl group in the Merck compound greatly reduces activity. In our case, in the case of enkephalinase, there is no additional subsite, S_1, for instance. We have, of course, prepared the analogue of the Merck compound, in the case of enkephalinase, and the first compound does not interact like thiorphan, for instance, because there is no additional S_1 binding site.

Professor Andrews
I agree that the basis for claiming that the compound is a transition state analogue originally was not strong. However, I would say that our studies of all those angiotensin-converting enzyme inhibitors, looking at the four binding groups – the benzyl, carbonyl, zinc-binding function and the carboxyl – relating them back to a proposed transition state structure, certainly suggest that they can all be regarded as transition state analogues.

9 General Discussion of Session I

CHAIRMAN: PROFESSOR TOMLINSON

Professor Tomlinson

I would like to focus on two general areas for discussion which are as follows:

1) The concept of drug targeting, which was so eloquently advocated by Professor Trouet − drug targeting, whether using a carrier or a conjugate system, and of course the pro-drug approach described by Professor Wermuth. Do they have a real significance in improving drug action? If they do have a real significance, I suppose the question that we may be able to ask is whether they are commercially viable, and do they have a real significance for drug design, in the classical sense that we know it?

2) Arising from a number of discussions, starting with Professor Marshall's, although computational chemistry (as he well proved) is a fact, can it be used rationally to design new drugs, does it still require a high degree of serendipity, and how can it be matched, for example, into the pharmacological receptor approach outlined by Professor Roques? I believe that some of Dr Wold's comments, and some of the latter comments by Professor Andrews will direct that discussion later.

First, the point about drug targeting. Are there any general points which we should raise? I am particularly intrigued by drug targeting because it is a specific pharmaceutical problem; it is an area where drug formulation meets drug design. That interface is a very exciting one for me personally, and one in which we are heavily involved in Amsterdam. Would Professor Trouet like to comment on the role of the pharmaceutical scientist − the formulation scientist − in the use of carrier molecules, particulate molecules, in particular perhaps the liposome systems, as carriers for drug targeting.

Professor Trouet

I agree that drug targeting is something in between drug formulation and drug design. But if we come back to the problem of cancer, for example, it is truly drug design because what hope have we of developing specific, selective anticancer drugs from what is known of the basic biochemical and molecular differences between a normal and a cancer cell? From what is known today, with the latest data on oncogenes and so on, there is no basic difference between a normal and a cancer cell. The hope today of developing the penicillin for cancer is zero. Drug design in cancer, therefore, in terms of developing a drug which would selectively act on tumour cells, and not on normal cells, is not a question at the moment of finding a compound, or of designing a compound, which will act at the receptor, at the molecular level, specific for a tumour cell.

We have potent chemical compounds which are able to interfere with some cellular mechanisms. The question is whether we can make use of some, perhaps antigenic or surface, properties of the cancer cells, selectively to direct to these cancer cells compounds which act in a general way.

I think, therefore, that drug targeting in cancer is drug design because there is no other way for the time being.

With regard to the question about liposomes, if a carrier is used, and if we want to send a drug to a given target cell, the first requirement needed for the carrier is that this carrier should not be taken up in a rather non-specific way by normal cells. Precisely the problem today with liposomes is that liposomes injected are taken up by the reticulo-endothelial system. If we want to send the drug to these cells, it is all right − and it has been done in the case of leishmaniasis, where antimonial drugs have been incorporated in liposomes, and have been shown to be very active. However, if we want to use liposomes as carriers, for example, to cancer cells, we first have to devise liposomes which are not taken up by the macrophages.

Professor Tomlinson
It seemed to me in the carrier field that we were putting old wine in new bottles, but it also seems to me that as that field of carrier technology is developing we are trying to marry the two together − the drug design and the drug formulation. A comment which was very prominent in the early days of the liposomes was that we were just trying to put an ordinary compound into a carrier to overcome its pharmacokinetic problems and toxicity effects. What Professor Trouet has shown is that, in fact, carriers can be designed at the same time as the new drugs are being developed. That is a very exciting viewpoint.

Dr Dearden
May I make a brief comment about one example in the field of pro-drugs, namely, the dipivaloyl derivative of epinephrine, which seems to me to be an example of a very interesting type of compound. That is, one which is applied more or less topically, being used for application to the eye in the treatment of glaucoma. Epinephrine itself is quite a polar compound. One *may* therefore assume that the receptor site demands a fairly polar compound.

On the other hand, because it is topical application, there are very few partitioning steps which the drug has to go through, and it can be shown theoretically that what is needed for best penetration in that circumstance is a high lipophilicity.

This example of Higuchi's, in which he stepped up the lipophilicity, increasing log P by something like two units, very neatly gets round both these problems. There is very rapid absorption to a topical receptor site and yet, because the pivaloyl groups cleave off, we are left with the polar drug which binds very well to the receptor. This probably accounts for the very high activity of the prodrug, something like 100-fold greater than that of epinephrine itself. That is a very neat example of a combined targeting and prodrug type of approach.

Dr Jolles

When we do drug design we expect, sooner or later, to have a drug to sell. To be slightly provocative, I would like to ask Professor Trouet if he feels that the very sophisticated molecules that he is building, with the protein, then a spacer arm, then a drug, are scientific gadgets or if they will be drugs sooner or later?

I feel that with regard to cancer, there is no problem about money – people can spend whatever they want, within certain limits. However, when we consider tropical diseases, or analgesics, very common drugs, does he not feel that the commercial aspects will be a limitation to the development of drug targeting? As I say, we have to come to this point in the designing of drugs, sooner or later.

Professor Trouet

I have first to answer as a scientist, and as someone interested in medicine. If I thought that I was talking only about gadgets, I would not have come to this meeting. We have to decide whether this concept is scientifically feasible and has any scientific value. This is our first aim, our first goal. We have to determine whether drug targeting is really possible, feasible and practicable.

The second question I would not answer as a scientist, but it has to be asked of the politicians, the philosophers. Let us suppose that this concept works, and that it is possible to prepare drugs and to target them selectively either to cancer cells or to protozoal infected cells. I agree that there will always be money to try to cure people with cancer. However, there are many more people suffering from tropical diseases. Having provided a scientific answer in that regard, I shall put the question to the politicians and to the people who govern this world. Are they ready to provide the means to solve these problems in their countries?

Professor Tomlinson

I think it is interesting that the Wellcome Foundation, which is not a typical drug company, has a liposome product which is about to be marketed for leishmaniasis – it is an antimony compound. They reckon that it is cost-effective, compared with a multiple emulsion or a fat emulsion, in that the dose regimen is once a week, instead of three times a day. When we start to look of these cost benefits, perhaps the proprietary view point can be answered.

Professor Trouet

I would like to add that although, of course, it looks at the moment as though the preparation of, for example, a daunorubicin tetrapeptide monoclonal antibody conjugate is very expensive, if it is proven scientifically that the concept is valid, I think that progress in the development of biotechnology and in chemistry will enable the cost to be improved for these preparations.

Professor Rabin

If it is possible to make a specific monoclonal antibody which binds to a tumour cell — that seems not unreasonable, in fact, for some lymphocytes in some particular situations — it does not seem to me that the drug end of it is needed any longer. All that is needed is the complement-fixing aspect. That may reduce the complications. Perhaps what is really needed is a collection of specific monoclonal antibodies.

However, there is one grave difficulty — that the monoclonal antibody would have to be raised for each case because it is most unlikely that there will be any overlap between one patient and another, in terms of the antibody they produce, which is actually the target for the system.

I think the difficulties are extremely grave because it means that the specific antibody would have to be raised for each individual patient. The practicality of that seems to me to be almost zero.

Professor Trouet

I agree with regard to the clonal antigens. If we want to develop anti-idiotypic antibodies, I agree. But these form only a small part. The concept will be worthwhile if it is possible to develop carriers with a broader spectrum. I do not think that it will be possible to have one carrier for all cancer cell types, but we can still hope that it will be possible to develop carriers for a given breast tumour. I am sure that carriers will not be found for all the tumour cells. It is our job to see what type of tumours can be attacked by this approach.

Professor Rabin

May I just say that I think the scientific basis of this should be given very high priority by all the funding authorities. Regardless of whether we can actually identify any practicality in the technology — and it looks very difficult at the moment — nevertheless, it is all we have currently because nothing else of which I know is rational.

Professor Tomlinson

Let us now turn to computational chemistry, perhaps computer graphics and molecular dynamics. At a number of meetings I have attended over the past three years I have seen the films and the 3-Ds, I have worn the glasses and have been impressed, I have used the Evans and Sutherland system and I have been even more impressed. The question now arises — and I am sure everyone has asked this question, perhaps in private — where is this going to take us? Professor Marshall's talk was very illustrative of that question. How do we start to match that sort of information to the receptor studies of Professor Roques, and the sort of studies discussed by Professor Andrews. Perhaps Professor Marshall would like to make a general comment.

Professor Marshall

What we are trying to do is to provide the medicinal chemists with a better tool. Exactly how it is used will obviously depend on the problem the medicinal chemist tackles, and on how science develops.

It seems to me that there is a convergence which, at least, I see through a glass darkly. Personally, I find trying to design inhibitors of enzymes much more tenable than going after receptor sites, primarily because of the reasons pointed out by Professor Andrews. There is a mechanism, and that mechanism possesses a geometry. We have the pharmacophore, if we want to think about it like that, because of the geometrical constraints of the chemistry that is going on. There is three-dimensional information now available on very many different types of enzymes. If we want to go for a redox enzyme, or something that uses NAD as a co-factor, there are nice examples — there are architectures, there are the beginnings of a three-dimensional background to use. If we then start trying to combine that possibility with trying to carry out QSAR in three-dimensions, and really use a lattice to look at properties, there is certainly a great potential — but it will only be when the medicinal chemist has the tools at his disposal that an impact will really be seen. As long as it stays in academia, everybody will dismiss it.

Professor Tomlinson

I think that is right. Certainly, a number of companies now are buying the systems, or buying time on systems. Would Professor Hansch like to comment on the systems?

Professor Hansch

I am very dedicated to graphics and its use, but I am not very optimistic about the use of graphics without the crystallography to start with — I mean crystallography of macromolecules, DNA, proteins or whatever we are working on. Our results indicate that even working with the crystallography of the enzyme, and QSAR, and making inhibitors, and everything else, there is still a long way to go before we really understand how ligands fit on the macromolecules and the perturbations that they cause.

One of the big problems that we see is that these macromolecules are much more flexible than physical chemists have led us to believe. That is now becoming generally accepted — that they are flexible, and that there is a great deal of movement. The question is how much? The more we look at the probes the more astonished we are how much movement there is.

The problem with the crystallography is that it is very slow in coming. We do not have many molecules for which the crystallography has been done. Until that comes along, we have to go along with what Professor Marshall is doing as best we can. That will call for much hard work, imagination and frustration — there will be a lot of disappointment in using that. But it is far better than nothing — there is no question about that.

Professor Andrews

To reinforce the last comment of Professor Hansch, I think that the role of calculations in designing new drugs can be divided into three broad categories.

First, to take the structure of existing drugs or related things like neurotrans-mitters, and to use an interpolative technique to try to find out what might be the particular structural requirements of all those drugs for activity. Originally, that was available in a two-dimensional way from the sort of techniques developed by Professor Hansch, and it is now becoming available three-dimensionally with Professor Marshall's approaches.

The second technique is to use a mechanism-based approach, in which the mechanism provides the guidance. That is what I tried to show in the transition state analogue case. Also, suicide inhibitors and so on can be used.

The difficulty with both these approaches is certainly the one just pointed out by Professor Hansch, that the receptor at which we are looking is an extremely flexible object, and it changes from one drug to another. Eventually, when we are trying to compare two or more drugs, there is the problem that we may be looking at compounds which actually bind to different receptor sites − although, of course, in the same protein. I think, therefore, that the third broad category in which the calculations will perhaps prove most valuable is in combination with crystal structures of receptors or enzymes, as they become available − admittedly, slowly. In designing analogues, we shall still have to do calculations which allow for the optimization both of the drug and of the enzyme at the same time to measure how good an interaction can be seen between those two structures. That is the only way in which it will be possible to use the crystal structure to design good inhibitors.

Professor Tomlinson
So, once again, a multidisciplinary approach − mixed with commonsense.

Dr Lunt
It does seem that one advantage that Professor Marshall's technique has over the design of specific analogues for the active site, or methods which involve studying the active site, is that it is probable that quite a lot of drug molecules do not actually act at the substrate site itself, but they modify that by acting at adjacent sites or even at sites remote from the active site itself, because of this flexibility − to which both Professor Hansch and Professor Andrews have just referred. It opens up that possibility, and the only way in which we can approach that is through some sort of empirical approach à la Professor Marshall in which the pharmacophore is fitted to the receptor site, whether or not it is the actual substrate site.

Professor Tomlinson
But is that not almost a semantic point? If it does not act at an active site, then it acts at an active site elsewhere.

Dr Lunt
Yes, but if, for example, a transition state analogue is designed, by definition, it is acting at the active site: the substrate site.

Professor Roques

Another problem in the measurement by an NMR technique, or by a calculation of conformational states in which molecules can bind to a receptor, is that if a receptor is a flexible molecule, there may be rotational change in the protein, for example. One conformational state of peptides, for instance, can be of very high energy, and in such conditions can be ignored. Because of the mutual interaction between the peptide and the receptor molecule, conformation in solution (seen by NMR, for instance, or calculated), can be induced in the active site of the receptor. The binding constant of protein to the receptor is very high, in the order of 10^{10}. Kinetically, it is possible to change the conformational states of a molecule like a peptide so that it assumes a very favourable or a very unfavourable conformation.

Professor Marshall

We have to realize that binding to proteins can cause breakage of carbon—carbon bonds. That goes on all the time. There is obviously a continuum with which we have to deal.

Certainly, one of the things about which we have felt very strongly is that we should look at a sufficient amount of conformational space, actually to examine those states which are probably without covalent cleavage, so that we get a good sampling of conformational space, and that we allow ourselves enough energy above the minima to do that. That is a very important point, and I think there are many reports in the literature where, if we look at the cases where it is known what bound states look like, they are not what is seen in isolation and not what is calculated as energy minima.

Certainly, in looking at the bound states of NAD, of which there are six or seven crystal structures, we see something not seen in NMR.

I agree that it is a problem. We have to look perhaps much more broadly than we would prefer. On the other hand, I think I shall come back to being very pragmatic about the whole subject. We are really dealing with levels of approximation. We have not spent much effort in trying to worry about potencies of compounds, but are much more interested in trying to define the stadium in which the game is being played, and perhaps what the game is that we are playing. As we try to become more sophisticated, and try to do things such as calculating binding affinities, it will be found that there are things like solvation, entropy and so on – the sort of things that we casually ignore or dismiss – which have to be taken into account. For a biochemist, somebody interested in biophysics, in protein structure and so on, these are really important issues.

As a medicinal chemist, I am not convinced that it will have a dramatic effect on me, on what I make at the bench next week. I am very schizoid – being a physical biochemist, on the one hand and worrying about things like that, and, on the other hand, facing the practical issue of what I need to address.

Dr Bost

In which direction does Professor Marshall think he will develop his system? He mentioned, for instance, solvation or entropy problems. What type of more accurate description of the molecule can be expected from his system at the moment?

Professor Marshall

We are collaborating with Dr Hagler, at the University California at San Diego, on molecular dynamics. We are very interested in the entropy problem, peptide conformations, solvation and that whole area, scientifically. It will be a long time before we know whether that will have a real impact in terms of drug design. Until we look − and look hard − it is pure speculation.

The area that I see to be the most efficient, in terms of practical utility, is the area of parameters. Getting good force field parameters, and knowing that we have energy values, and being confident about geometries and so on is fairly trivial for hydrocarbons and a few other things, but if we get esoteric (and most of us are getting esoteric with chemistry), then being confident, and knowing how to get good parameters still remains something of a problem. That is an area in which we plan − we hope − to evaluate some quantum approaches.

Session II

10 The New Look to QSAR

C. HANSCH and J.M. BLANEY*

*Seaver Chemistry Laboratory, Pomona College,
Claremont, California 91711 USA
* School of Pharmacy, Department of Pharmaceutical Chemistry, University of California,
San Francisco, California 94143, USA*

Introduction

The subject of this meeting, "Drug Design: Fact or Fantasy?", is the result of greatly increased discussion about the *possibilities* for drug design. Obviously we have not reached the point where one can sit down at a computer and work out the structure of a novel heart drug. To many of those who have spent a good part of their lives trying, with very rare success, to find new drugs, the casual use of the term "drug design" may seem naive and even egotistical. They know all too well that drugs are not designed — they are discovered. Luck always plays a major role in the finding of a truly novel drug (Hansch, 1974). However, the fact that drug design techniques are crude and often unreliable does not mean that we can give up developing a science of drug design. Drug design did not arrive with computers, it has always been attempted. Style in drug design at any point in time is determined by two factors: *concepts about the cause of disease* and *the level of accumulated experience.*

Many ancients operated under the assumption that disease was caused by evil spirits entering the body so it is not surprising that research in those days involved finding agents to drive out the spirits. In the light

DRUG DESIGN: FACT OR FANTASY
ISBN 0.12.388180.3

of this philosophy it is interesting to consider an Egyptian drug in use about 2000 BC for inflamed eyes. The drug was composed by taking equal parts of myrrh, cypress flowers, citron pips, Great Protector's seed, white oil, copper oxide, antimony, gazelle droppings and oryx dung and placing them in water over night. The concoction was filtered through cloth before use (Partington, 1935). It seems clear that a good deal of design went into this drug. Sugar coating (myrrh, cypress flowers) was part of accumulated experience 4000 years ago as was the soothing effect of white oil. Of course copper and antimony salts are toxic to microorganisms and this too may well have been recognized long before 2000 BC. The exotic dung (the best is none too good) was probably presumed to be effective in driving out the evil spirits. This crude mixture, which was likely the end product of many many years of trying out all kinds of wild and desperate means for treating disease, may have had considerable benefit.

Modern philosophy about the nature of disease began to develop about 100 years ago when in 1865 Pasteur made his magnificent demonstrations of the presence (and later the importance) of microorganisms. Lister, on learning of Pasteur's ideas asked a chemist friend for a suggestion of a chemical which might kill bacteria (drive out the evil spirits). Anderson's suggestion of carbolic acid paid off beautifully. Phenol had been used by the Egyptians in embalming and at the time of Anderson was used to preserve railroads ties from decay. Philosophy and accumulated experience came together to "design" a new drug. Phenol soon greatly increased one's chances of not dying of infection in hospitals. It was a dangerous drug because of its great toxicity. The famous organic chemist Kolbe, set out to change this by converting phenol to salicylic acid (a nice synthetic procedure he had just discovered). He mistakenly believed that salicylic acid slowly reverted into the phenol and CO_2 from which it was made. Crude experiments showed salicylic acid to be much less toxic than phenol and use on patients was soon started. Patients felt much better taking salicylic acid, but prolongation of life did not follow. It was then discovered that salicylic acid was an analgesic and fever reducer and in addition it could be very irritating to the stomach. Drug modification by way of acetylation produced aspirin. By 1900, the rapid development of organic chemistry was supplying a hoard of new substances, dwarfing anything the Egyptians could have imagined, for testing against disease. In fact the possibilities became essentially infinite.

Ehrlich's monumental achievement in 1909 of the discovery of a specific cure for the scourge of syphilis had a profound affect on drug research. Ehrlich and his colleagues made over 600 compounds in an attempt to find a cure for trypanosomiasis. Although the 606th compound was inactive against trypanosomes, Ehrlich's co-worker, S. Hata, decided to try it on syphilis because of the superficial similarities between trypanosomes and spirochetes. It worked and Ehrlich was showered with honours including the Nobel prize. The lesson from this research was that simply by testing enough compounds one could eventually find a cure for any disease. While this "random" screening of new chemicals led to the discovery of many important new drugs (e.g. the sulphas) we have reached the point where it is becoming much less effective.

The most convincing demonstration that random screening plus "systematic" modification of the active compounds uncovered will not always work has been made by the National Cancer Institute. In the 1950s the Institute undertook the screening of every and any organic compound it could obtain. By now about 400,000 chemicals have been tested and although many compounds with various degrees of antitumour activity have been developed none can be said to cure cancer. The many billions of dollars spent on synthesizing, animal testing and a huge number of clinical trials have been instructive in many ways. One of the most important lessons is that to find an agent highly selective for tumours with modest toxicity to normal cells calls for much more sophisticated science.

Until recently drug research has been dominated largely by organic chemists and pharmacologists, but now with the great advances of science in many fields I believe we are at the point of an explosive modification of our methods. The incredibly rapid advances in biochemistry, molecular biology, theoretical chemistry and computers along with the accumulated experience of the past 100 years must give drug research directors some sleepless nights. There are so many expensive avenues to explore that even with budgets in hundreds of millions of dollars it is no easy task placing one's bets. Picking the right approach in the search for a new drug is still largely a matter of faith.

I would like to consider drug design from the organic chemist's viewpoint. The seedlings for today's drug design began to sprout about the time of Ehrlich's famous work. The independent observations of Meyer and Overton that in a rough way the narcotic potency of simple neutral organic compounds parallels their lipophilicity (as defined by oil/water partition coefficients) was the beginning of a line of thinking which has resulted in our appreciation of the enormous importance of the hydrophobic interaction in biology. At about this same time the so-called English school of organic chemistry began to take an interest in the mechanisms of organic reactions (Ingold, 1969). By the 1930s the study of organic reactions had become rather highly developed although many of the concepts (such as inductive, resonance and steric effects) could only be expressed in qualitative terms. A major turning point in mechanistic organic chemistry just at the outbreak of World War II in 1940, was the publication of the first edition of "Physical Organic Chemistry" by L.P. Hammett (Hammett, 1970). Although the book treated many aspects of physical organic chemistry its greatest achievement was the introduction of the σ constants as a quantitative measure of the electronic effect of substituents on aromatic rings on reaction rates and equilibria. Hammett's use of numbers and statistical analysis began the conversion (which may never be completed) of organic chemistry to an exact science. It is hard to over-estimate the value of Hammett's conceptual breakthrough — the use of a model system (ionization of benzoic acids) to develop the numerical σ constant scale. Hammett's student, Taft, quickly grasped the importance of the concept and devised a numerical scale E_s for the steric effects of substituents (Taft, 1956). He also showed how the electronic effect could be factored into two numerical scales one for the inductive and the other for resonance effects of substituents. Regression analysis could now be employed to delineate the relative importance of these effects.

Shortly after this in the early sixties, the Pomona College group combined Hammett's idea for formulating numerical scales from equilibrium constants with Meyer and Overton's operational definition of lipophilicity via octanol/water partition coefficients to define a hydrophobicity scale for substituents (π) as well as whole molecules (log P) (Hansch *et al.*, 1962; Hansch, 1969). With the great expansion of the use of large computers which commenced in 1965 with the advent of the IBM 360 series, the stage was set for attacking SAR as a multidimensional problem. It is at this point that the *possibilities* for drug design took a great leap forward. The combination of computerized regression analysis (not widely available before 1960) and statistics allowed the *objective* testing of all kinds of ideas from physical organic and structural chemistry. Data on hundreds or thousands of compounds, impossible for any chemist to keep in mind, could now be manipulated with the greatest of ease. We are only at the very beginning of the effective use of computers in attacking the horrendously complex SAR problem, but at this point one can no longer take the comfortable view that the biochemical processes evoked by a set of congeners are too complex to be treated mathematically. Multidimensional statistical techniques, when coupled with well thought out physicochemical parameters and molecular graphics, are bound to have a large influence in drug development. The old approach, which was in effect doing regression analysis by the seat of one's pants, is no longer tenable.

The general expression below gives the premise upon which medicinal chemists have operated qualitatively for many years and with which we have made considerable progress quantitatively in the past two decades.

$$\text{Biological Activity} = f(\text{physicochemical properties})$$

The problem of rationalizing the biological activity of a set of congeneric drugs with their physical properties could not have been seriously attacked before the general use of computers in the early sixties.

Now that we are well into the business of formulating mathematical models for biochemical structure–activity relationships (QSAR) it becomes pertinent to ask why there are not a variety of cases of the design of commercial drugs based on computerized approaches. My own view of this is that only a very few groups have yet spent enough time getting an in-depth understanding of just how to use QSAR in drug design. It is easy enough to build all sorts of computer generated models, but these models are no better than the data on which they are based. Friends in the drug companies tell me that it is simply not possible to get accurate test data from complex biological test systems for a variety of reasons. Chief among these is the high cost and the lack of faith that better quality data would provide added insight into the SAR.

To get the most out of QSAR we need to organize the results of the last 20 years into a coherent structure which will enable many more people to enter the field with a reasonable investment of time. Of course, this is a job for the universities, very few of which have people capable of attempting it. I believe that at least another decade will pass before a significant number of schools will have first class studies in QSAR and it will take another decade before their students will produce the kind of effect I visualize computers will have in drug design.

The central problem in drug research is that of the selective control of biochemical processes. For most of the drugs now in use this selectivity was not understood at the time of their discovery but only became evident much later if at all. QSAR is a method with exciting possibilities for understanding and exploiting the selective control of biochemical processes. So far, relatively few academic laboratories are going about the systematic development of QSAR. Too many researchers are content to derive some kind of an equation with a reasonable correlation coefficient and let things go at that stage. In fact, much basic research is needed which is not very close to the actual making of new drugs and hence not likely to be done by researchers in drug companies.

One of the best places to develop our ideas about how drugs interact with receptors is with the QSAR of enzymes. My thinking about this subject has been greatly influenced by the pioneering work of Baker (1967) and Hitchings (Hitchings and Smith, 1979). Enzymes constitute the best studied macromolecular receptors for drugs for which the detailed structures are known. X-ray crystallography has provided us with the three-dimensional structures of a number of important enzymes and no doubt the structures of many others will be done before long. The techniques and promises of the X-ray crystallography of macromolecules have become so promising that at least three drug companies now support such groups. Others will likely follow their lead.

The crystallography of organic compounds binding to nucleic acids is also beginning to attract attention and this too offers benefits for the medicinal chemist (Quigley *et al.*, 1980; Tsai *et al.*, 1977). With the increasing evidence that drugs may produce their effects by interaction with DNA the X-ray crystallography of synthetic fragments of DNA should enable us to understand such interaction mechanisms.

A surprising approach to the three-dimensional structure of macromolecules is the use of high resolution NMR coupled with distance geometry analysis which is being pioneered by Wuthrich and his co-workers (Braun *et al.*, 1981; Brown *et al.*, 1982). It now appears that their approach may be able to deduce the structures of small enzymes in solution.

The last two decades have seen a much greater interest in enzymes develop among medicinal chemists. The Journal of Biochemical Pharmacology, for example, started publishing in 1957 and in 1960 published 505 pages. In 1980 it published 3346 much larger pages. In 1960 the Journal of Medicinal Chemistry published 48 papers 5 of which dealt with a total of three different enzymes. In 1980, the journal published 297 papers 38 of which were devoted to 25 different enzymes. Six of the papers were devoted to dihydrofolate reductase. The quest for greater selectivity seems to be going more and more to the molecular level. In short, the point of view of our group is that X-ray crystallography, QSAR and molecular graphics offer the best opportunity for a more fundamental understanding of selectivity as well as providing some insight into the means microorganisms have for developing resistance.

One of the more difficult problems those working with enzymic SAR have had to contend with is that of disentangling the binding parameters for ligands binding with macromolecules. The recent breakthroughs in colour three-dimensional computerized graphics are going to be of enormous help in solving some of these problems (Langridge *et al.*, 1981; Feldman *et al.*, 1978). Our first studies with enzymic SAR and molecular graphics have been encouraging (Smith *et al.*, 1982; Hansch *et al.*, 1982; Li *et al.*, 1982; Blaney *et al.*, 1982).

Papain SAR

The hydrolase papain is a useful enzyme on which to sharpen some of the tools of the QSAR paradigm (Unger, 1980). Its mechanism of action is similar to the serine hydrolases, however, it employs the SH moiety of cysteine residue in the formation of the tetrahedral intermediate in the cleavage of esters. The following two classes of esters yielded the corresponding QSAR (Smith *et al.*, 1982; Hansch *et al.*, 1977b).

$$\log 1/K_m = 1.01\,\pi + 1.46 \qquad [1]$$
$$n = 16, r = 0.981, s = 0.165$$

$$\log 1/K_m = 1.03\,\pi'_3 + 0.57\,\sigma + 0.61\,MR_4 + 3.80 \qquad [2]$$
$$n = 25, r = 0.907, s = 0.208$$

In these expressions K_m is the Michaelis constant which we assume to be an approximate binding constant, n represents the number of data points on which the QSAR is based, r is the correlation coefficient and s is the standard deviation.

Equation 1 is a simple model which rationalizes 96% of the variance in $\log 1/K_m$ for 16 methyl hippurates with substituents in the 3- or 4-position binding to papain.

Except for a 3,5-di-NO_2 analogue the other derivatives bore either a single 3- or 4-substituent. The slope of 1 for Eq. 1 suggests that the hippurates partition on to papain in the same way they partition between octanol/water (Hansch and Leo, 1979). Hence, one assumes that Y is more or less completely desolvated in binding to papain and that the region into which Y falls must be made up of largely hydrophobic residues. Equation 2 is a much more complicated expression which explains only 82% of the variance in log $1/K_m$. In this equation π'_3 means that only the hydrophobic constant for the more hydrophobic of the two meta substituents of (2) is used. For the other meta substituent π'_3 is set equal to zero. Only by making such an assumption could a reasonable correlation equation be derived. The logic behind the assumption was that the hydrophobic binding of one meta substituent placed the other meta substituent in the extraenzymic aqueous phase. The positive coefficient with the σ term shows that electron withdrawing substituents favour formation of the E_s complex, one expects and finds that withdrawal of electrons favours the approach of the electron rich SH group. The variable MR_4 applies only to 4-substituents. Since molar refractivity (MR) is primarily a measure of bulk (Hansch and Leo, 1979) the positive coefficient with this term brings out the point that the larger X_4 is the better the binding. However, this is not a hydrophobic effect since MR and π are reasonably orthogonal and the data do not correlate with π_4.

Equation 2 tells us to look for a hydrophobic pocket for X_3 and polar space for the interaction of X_4.

In the first stereo view* (Plate I) we see a composite molecule made up of structures (1) and (2) binding to the active site of a model of papain constructed from coordinates of papain obtained by Drenth (Drenth *et al.*, 1970). The surface of the enzyme has been colour coded red for hydrophobic space and blue for polar space. It is immediately apparent that Y binds in a large red hydrophobic cleft easily able to accommodate the largest Y studied (4-O-n-C_4H_9). In this model X_3 falls naturally into a hydrophobic pocket forcing X_5 into the aqueous phase.

It has been assumed, since π correlates binding in hydrophobic space, that when π and MR are orthogonal and the correlation is with MR hydrophobic space cannot be involved and binding in polar space is implied. In Plate I X_4 is pointing toward a blue bulge which is the surface of the ϵ-NH_2 of Gln-142. Of course this amide moiety on the surface of papain would be hydrated so that its effective size should be larger than shown in Plate I. The flexible -$CH_2CH_2\overset{\displaystyle O}{\overset{\displaystyle \|}{C}}NH_2$ of the Gln-142 appears to function as an adjustable buttress working against X_4 helping to position the esters in the E_s complex for hydrolysis.

Plate II shows both ligand and enzyme with their respective surfaces

---

* A "stereo-viewer", suitable for use with Plate I, has been designed by Professor F. Vögtle and distributed by Verlag Chemie (obtainable from the Royal Society of Chemistry in England).

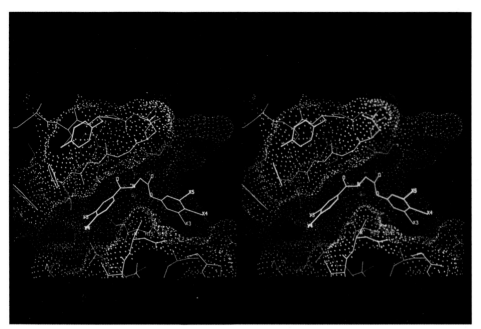

PLATE I

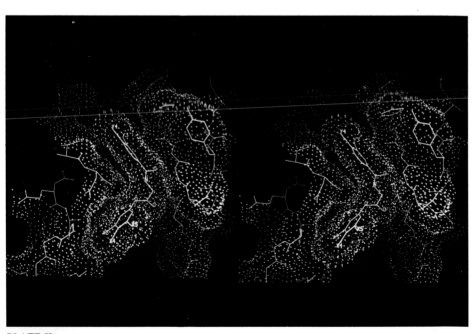

PLATE II

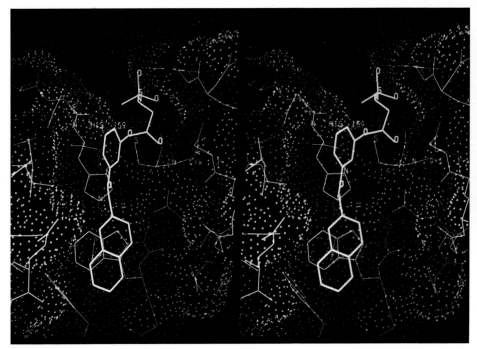

PLATE III

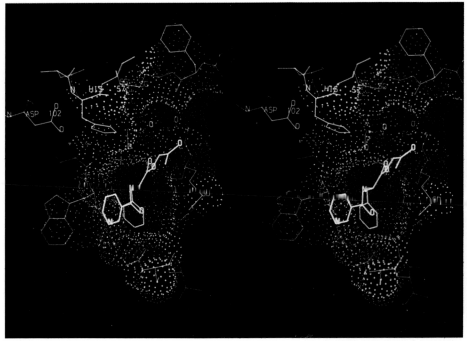

PLATE IV

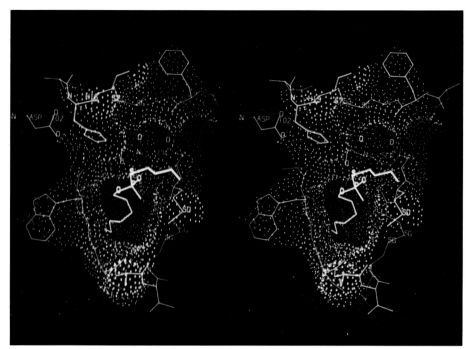

PLATE V

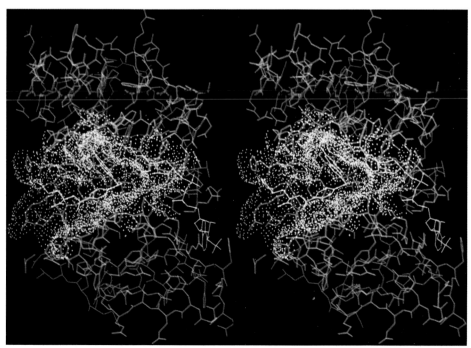

PLATE VI

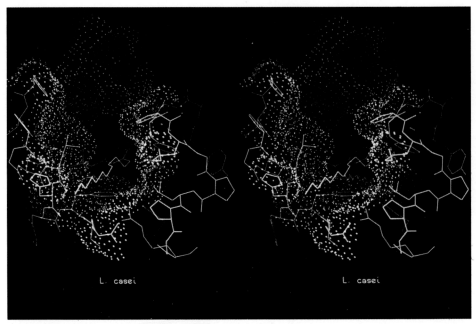

PLATE VII

with that of the ligand in green. The impressive closeness of fit reminds one of the "lock-and-key" concept of enzyme-ligand interaction. Water associated with X_3 would have to be completely desolvated in the formation of such a complex.

From the graphics studies it was estimated that the largest group which would fit in the X_3 binding site would be 3-*t*-butyl and that 3-C_6H_5 would be too large to be well predicted by Eq. 2.

Because of the limited aqueous solubility of congeners (2) it was decided in extending the study to select the more soluble parent structure (3).

3

From the papain hydrolysis of variations of (3) Eq. 3 was derived (Carotti *et al.*).

$$\log 1/K_m = 0.61 \, \pi'_3 + 0.55 \, \sigma + 0.46 \, MR_4 + 2.00 \qquad [3]$$
$$n = 32, r = 0.945, s = 0.178$$

Equation 3 was a shock to us. Although the agreement between the σ terms of Eqs 2 and 3 is excellent and the MR_4 terms are rather close, the coefficients with the π terms are definitely different. As expected the 3-*t*-butyl analogue was well fit, but the 3-phenyl congener was only a little less active than predicted by Eq. 3. This called for testing still larger groups and we were quite surprised to find that 3-$OCH_2C_6H_5$, 3-$OCH_2C_6H_4$-4'-Cl and 3-OCH_2-2'-naphthyl were all well fit by Eq. 3, although they obviously can not fit into the hydrophobic pocket suggested in Plate I. Our present hypothesis for rationalizing the model of Eq. 3 is shown in Plate III. The phenyl ring has now been rotated so as to place the -OCH_2-2'-naphthyl moiety out over a hydrophobic surface of a tryptophan residue. Presumably in this mode of hydrophobic interaction only the surface of say 3-OCH_2-2'-naphthyl adjacent to the protein would be desolvated. The other side of the substituent would remain in contact with the aqueous phase. This would account for a coefficient with the π term in Eq. 3 about half the size of that in Eq. 2.

Equations 2 and 3 were formed from data consisting mostly of 3- or

4-monosubstituted congeners. However, polysubstituted derivatives are well fit. Equation 3 fits the 3, 4, 5-trichloro analogue quite well. In order to give Eq. 3 a more rigorous test a derivative, 3-t-butyl-4-NO$_2$ predicted to be more active than any yet studied, was synthesized and tested. It was fitted beautifully by Eq. 3.

The reason for the different binding mode for congeners (3) compared to congeners (2) is by no means clear. It is probably related to the hydrophobic character of the two different anchoring groups: NHSO$_2$CH$_3$, NHCOC$_6$H$_5$. The benzoyl group fits nicely into the large hydrophobic cleft and strongly promotes binding. The highly polar sulphonamide is not so well accommodated so that these congeners are not well positioned to make contact with the hydrophobic pocket available for 3-X of (2).

The results with Eqs 2 and 3 show just how tricky ligand binding to macromolecules can be and how even with good data, good QSAR and high level graphics one can be quite surprised in testing new congeners. This is an old story to medicinal chemists. The message in these results is that at the molecular level one can understand and adjust one's strategy to take advantage of such information. With the best results from cell culture or whole animals it would be difficult if not impossible to deduce the cause of unexpected interactions even with the imaginative use of modern graphics. QSAR has a unique role to play in increasing our understanding of ligand–receptor interactions as of course do X-ray crystallography and graphics.

Chymotrypsin SAR

A quite different QSAR-crystallography-graphics case comes from the study of another hydrolase, chymotrypsin (Hansch *et al.*, 1977; Grieco *et al.*, 1979; Silipo *et al.*, 1979). One sees in Plate IV and Plate V, of the active site of chymotrypsin, a different receptor geometry. The QSAR of Eq. 4 and 5 have been derived for acylaminoacid esters (4).

4a   4b

Structure (4a) shows the L-form with the three R groups binding in p_1, p_2 and p_3 space of the enzyme. Structure (4b) suggests how the D-form of these esters might bind to the same receptor.

The QSAR of Eq. 4 correlates a set of 71 esters (4a) interacting with chymotrypsin (Hansch *et al.*, 1977a).

$$\log 1/K_m = 1.09\,MR_2 + 0.80\,MR_1 + 0.52\,MR_3 + 0.63I + 1.26\,\sigma^*$$
$$- 0.057\,MR_1.MR_2.MR_3 - 1.61 \qquad [4]$$
$$n = 71, r = 0.979, s = 0.332$$

The subscribed MR terms refer to the R_s of (4). The indicator variable I takes the value of 1 when R_2 = isopropyl(valine) and σ^* is associated with the leaving group $-OR_3$. Its positive coefficient shows that as with papain formation of the E_s complex is favoured by electron withdrawing substituents. The cross product term shows that when two very large groups are present or when three moderately large groups are present the result is poorer binding. Up to the point where the $MR_1.MR_2.MR_3$ terms become significant binding is largely controlled by the molar refractivity of MR of the three substituents. Using π in Eq. 4 yields much poorer correlations even though there is considerable collinearity between π_1 and MR_1, π_2 and MR_2 and π_3 and MR_3. In order to more clearly delineate the role of MR, 13 new variations of (4a) were synthesized in which R_1 and R_2 were held constant (R_2 = CH_3, R_1 = nicotinyl) but wide variation was included in R_3 in such a way that MR_3 and π_3 were reasonably orthogonal. The additional results were refit along with the earlier data to produce Eq. 5 (Grieco *et al.*, 1979).

$$\log 1/K_m = 1.13\,MR_2 + 0.77\,MR_1 + 0.47\,MR_3 \quad 0.56I + 1.35\,\sigma^*$$
$$- 0.055\,MR_1.MR_2.MR_3 - 1.64 \qquad [5]$$
$$n = 84, r = 0.977, s = 0.333$$

The parameters of Eq. 5, including the goodness of fit, agree well with Eq. 4. Since binding by R_3 is well correlated by MR but badly correlated by π it was concluded that p_3 space is polar. Plate IV shows the model of the active site of chymotrypsin with the substrate where R_2 = $CH_2C_6H_5$, R_1 = C_5H_4N, R_3 = CH_2COCH_3. The benzyl moiety is in the so-called hydrophobic hole and the nicotinoyl portion falls on a rather broad surface which is half blue and half red. It seems likely that parameterization of R_1 for binding in this region may be difficult. Although Eq. 5 correlates such binding well, the variation in R_1 is not great. While 12 different examples of R_1 have been studied few highly hydrophilic substituents were included.

The character of ϱ_3 space where the OCH_2COCH_3 moiety binds is largely hydrophilic (blue). The two labels O locate two tightly bound water molecules showing that polar groups are favoured in this region. Toward the right of p_3 space there is a large red hydrophobic area to which long flexible hydrophobic chains could bind. The OCH_2COCH_3 unit has been arranged so that the CH_3 group is near this region. In the upper left side of the p_3 region there is an $-S-S-$ linkage colour coded yellow because of the uncertainty as to whether it should be classified as hydrophobic or hydrophilic. This group appears to show no preference for either phase. For instance log P for CH_3CH_3 is 1.81 and log P for CH_3SSCH_3 is almost identical (1.77). It seems likely that substituent binding to $-SS-$ would be better correlated by MR than by π because of the unpaired electrons on S.

About p_2 space we can make no firm statement from QSAR studies since the R_2 groups so far studied are such that π and MR are almost perfectly collinear.

The D esters (4b) yield the QSAR of Eq. 6.

$$\log 1/K_m = 0.47MR_2 + 1.38MR_1 + 1.83I + 2.76 \qquad [6]$$
$$n = 15, r = 0.993, s = 0.267$$

In this expression I takes the value of 1 when $R_3 = C_6H_4\text{-}4'\text{-}NO_2$ and 0 for $R_3 = $ Me. Only this limited type of variation was studied for R_3. Note that the size of the coefficients with MR_2 and MR_1 in Eq. 6 are the reverse of Eq. 5 suggesting the "wrong way" binding as shown in structure (4b). The graphics models of chymotrypsin show a large hydrophobic hole and rather open areas of p_1 and p_3 space so that binding does not seem to be highly restricted.

The graphics model in Plate V illustrates the binding of a set of phosphorus esters (5) to chymotrypsin (Silipo *et al.*, 1979).

$$p_3$$

$$SR_3$$
$$|$$
$$P\cdots\cdots O$$
$$R_2O \diagup \quad \diagdown CH_3$$

$$p_2 \qquad\qquad p_1$$

5

The QSAR for these inhibitors is displayed in Eq. 7.

$$\log 1/K_i = 1.42MR_{OR_2} + 0.35MR_{R_3} + 1.21\sigma^* - 3.30 \log (\beta.10^{MR_{OR_2}} + 1) - 5.18 \qquad [7]$$
$$n = 40, r = 0.981, s = 0.253, \text{ ideal } MR_{OR_2} = 3.75$$

K_i in this expression is the bimolecular rate constant for phosphorylation of chymotrypsin. The arrangement of the ester (5) in enzymic space is similar to that of the esters (4). The leaving group SR_3 is placed near p_3 space and the most hydrophobic group R_2 is placed into p_2 space (hydrophobic hole). Despite the fact that the geometry of the P in (5) is different from that of the central C in (4) the coefficients of Eq. 7 are rather similar to those of Eq. 5. The coefficients of $1.42 MR_{OR^2}$ is a little higher than $1.13 MR_2$ and that of $0.35 MR_{R_3}$ is slightly lower than $0.47 MR_3$. The σ terms are in good agreement. Not enough bulk was built in the variations of (5) to justify the use of the triple cross product term of Eqs 4 and 5, however, it was necessary to use the bilinear model of Kubinyi and Kehrhahn (1978) to account for the poor fit of the large OR_2 groups in p_2 space. The ideal MR of 3.75 corresponds to a group the size $O(CH_2)_7CH_3$. Although the OR_2 group in Plate V is placed in the large hole of p_2 the $SCH_2CH_2CH_2CH_3$ moiety has been arranged so that it interacts mainly with red hydrophobic space near p_3. The methyl group which is constant in this set of compounds is placed near a hydrophobic wall. It does not have the size or right geometry to contact what we have considered as p_1 space in Plate IV.

Since variations in R_2 and R_3 of (5) are almost completely limited to CH_2 groups MR and π are collinear. MR has been used in Eq. 7 instead of π for easy comparison with Eq. 5.

Plates IV and V show a receptor with a large binding hole which can accept a phenyl or indolyl moiety with room to spare. The p_1 area is also large and obstruction free so that large variation in the size of R_1 is also possible. Even the catalytically important p_3 area which contains the essential serine attacking group is rather open. Thus, from this model it is easy to understand why chymotrypsin can operate on such a wide variety of substrates (Hansch *et al.*, 1977). There is a limit, however, in its ability to accept on equal terms substrates which have too much bulk in R_1, R_2 and R_3 and this necessitates the triple cross product term in Eq. 5. Whether this is the best way to account for lack of bulk tolerance needs further investigation. One can also fit the data well using $\Sigma(MR_{1,2,3})^2$ or the bilinear model.

Dihydrofolate Reductase SAR

An enzyme of great interest to medicinal chemists is dihydrofolate reductase (DHFR). A number of its inhibitors have found use in cancer chemotherapy (methotrexate, aminopterin, Baker's antifols) as well as bacterial chemotherapy (trimethoprim, tetroxoprim). The extensive X-ray crystallography being done on this enzyme from various sources by Kraut, Matthews and their colleagues at the University of California in San Diego (Matthews *et al.*, 1979; Matthews *et al.*, 1978; Volz *et al.*, 1982) is opening up the possibility for the most sophisticated kind of drug design. The graphics models in this report are based on coordinates obtained from their laboratory. Ideally one would like to study the action of inhibitors as prospective drugs on purified human enzyme and then on enzyme from the pathological cells of interest. The QSAR from these systems could then be used to design drugs with a known high therapeutic index. Equations 8–11 compare the inhibitory actions of triazines (6) on human and bacterial (*L. casei*) DHFR.

6

Inhibition of Human DHFR by 4-X-(6) (Hathaway *et al.*).

$$\log 1/K_i = 0.78\,\pi'_4 - 0.78\log(\beta.10^{\pi'4} + 1) + 1.26I - 0.88\nu + 5.83 \quad [8]$$
$$n = 35,\ r = 0.953,\ s = 0.361,\ \pi_0 = 3.43$$

Inhibition of Human DHFR by 3-X-(6) (Hathaway *et al.*).

$$\log 1/K_i = 1.07\,\pi'_3 - 1.10\log(\beta.10^{\pi'3} + 1) + 0.50I + 0.82\,\sigma + 6.07 \quad [9]$$
$$n = 60,\ r = 0.890,\ s = 0.308,\ \pi_0 = 1.84$$

Inhibition of *L. casei* DHFR by 4-X-(6) (Hansch *et al.*).

$$\log 1/K_i = 0.44\,\pi'_4 - 0.65\log(\beta.10^{\pi'4} + 1) - 0.90\nu + 0.69I + 4.67 \quad [10]$$
$$n = 35,\ r = 0.900,\ s = 0.420,\ \pi_0 = 4.53$$

Inhibition of *L. casei* DHFR by 3-X-(6) (Hansch *et al.*).

$$\log 1/K_i = 0.83\,\pi'_3 - 0.91\log(\beta.10^{\pi'3} + 1) + 0.71I + 4.00 \quad [11]$$
$$n = 38,\ r = 0.961,\ s = 0.244,\ \pi_0 = 2.69$$

The inhibitors have been split into two groups; those substituted in the 4-position and those substituted in the 3-position of (6). All of the equations are based on the Kubinyi bilinear model (Kubinyi and Kehrhahn, 1978). The π' symbol refers to substituents of the type -ZCH$_2$C$_6$H$_4$Y or -CH$_2$ZC$_6$H$_4$-Y where Z may be O, S, SO, or NH. For these substituents changes in Y do not produce significant changes in

K_i, hence it was assumed that Y does not contact the enzyme. All other substituents take the normal π values. The indicator variable I take the value of 1 for substituents 3- and 4-Z-$CH_2C_6H_4$-Y and 3- and 4-$CH_2ZC_6H_4$-Y for Eqs 8, 9, and 10. For Eq. 11 only moieties of the type -CH_2Z-C_6H_4-Y are parameterized with a 1. These benzyl moieties have an important and specific enhancing power on the binding of triazines which is almost always seen regardless of the type of DHFR. In the case of the human DHFR there is a marked difference between the coefficients with I in Eqs 8 and 9. The effect is much more important with 4- substituents. With *L. casei* DHFR 3- and 4- substituents behave in identical fashion for substituents of the type -$CH_2ZC_6H_5$ but differ for substituents of the type -$ZCH_2C_6H_5$.

The 3-X-triazines (Eq. 9) are different in that a σ term is significant. One might be inclined to view this as an artifact since it does not occur with 4- substituents. However it does appear in other equations based on results from bovine and murine enzyme (Guo *et al.*, 1981). The only apparent explanation for this is that 3-X-triazines bind in a slightly different way from 4 so that a lower electron density on the 5-phenyl moiety favours binding.

The greatest difference between the human and the *L. casei* equation is in the intercepts. The intercept is a measure of the intrinsic activity in the two systems at least for the 3-X-triazine and *L. casei* where the slope of the π term is close to that of the two human equations. The lower slope of the π term in Eq. 10 means that for lipophilic congeners one cannot make such a comparison. Although Eqs 8 and 10 are not parallel the 4-X-triazines are even less active with *L. casei* DHFR than the 3 when compared to their activity with human DHFR. The parameter v is Charton's steric parameter (Charton, 1977) which is similar to Taft's E_s constant, however, more v are available than E_s values. The negative sign with this parameter in both Eqs 8 and 10 for 4-X-triazines brings out a deleterious steric effect at the 4- position not present in 3-X-triazines. In the case of *L. casei* DHFR study of the graphics models clearly shows the 4-X substituents run into Phe-49. Although the sequence of the human enzyme has not yet been completed there must be a residue comparable to Phe-49 in *L. casei* causing almost exactly the same steric effect (compare coefficients of v).

Although we do not as yet have X-ray crystallographic data on human DHFR such data is available for *L. casei* DHFR. Plate VI shows the graphics model of all of the *L. casei* DHFR backbone (in blue) with the active site region covered with a red surface in which methotrexate (MTX) (green) is residing. This model was constructed from the co-ordinates of the ternary complex (NADPH-DHFR-MTX) supplied to us by D.A. Matthews and J. Kraut of the University of California at

San Diego. The outline of the NADPH is coloured yellow. The surface of the active site occupies a large part of the whole enzyme and would appear considerably larger if a surface was also placed on the NADPH binding site. DHFR is an efficiently built enzyme with what would appear to be a minimum number of amino acid residues not involved directly in the active site.

Plate VII shows the *L. casei* DHFR with $3\text{-O(CH}_2)_{10}\text{CH}_3$-triazine in it. This model was constructed from the coordinates used to construct Plate VI. The MTX was replaced with the triazine with nitrogen atoms of the triazine superimposed on the positions occupied by the corresponding atoms of MTX. The long alkyl chain has been placed along the red hydrophobic floor of the enzyme. The QSAR results do not support this binding mode for 3-X-triazines but suggest that it is reasonable for 4-X-triazines. The π_0 value for 2-X-triazines is only 2.7 (equivalent to $\text{O(CH}_2)_5\text{CH}_3$) while π_0 for 4-X-triazines is 4.5 (equivalent to $\text{O(CH}_2)_8\text{CH}_3$). The lengthy hydrophobic floor can accommodate 9 to 10 atoms. If the long 4-OR groups bind along this floor then they would be open to solvent on one side since the cleft is rather wide. Desolvation would not be complete on binding which would explain the low coefficient of about 0.5 with π in Eq. 10.

Another hypothesis is necessary for the 3-X-triazines. If we postulate that these bind above the floor between the two red bulges seen in the middle of Plate VII then desolvation would be complete and the binding pocket would be considerably smaller. This would account not only for the slope of π near 1 in Eq. 11, and the low π_0 value but also for the fact that in groups of the type $\text{-CH}_2\text{ZC}_6\text{H}_4\text{-Y}$ or $\text{-ZCH}_2\text{C}_6\text{H}_4\text{-Y}$ πY has been arbitrarily set to zero. In this model Y would not be able to reach the hydrophobic floor but would project into aqueous space.

There is one difficulty with the above model and that is the fact that πY has also been set to zero for such groups in the 4-X-triazines. One could get around this problem by suggesting that for these special phenyl groups which appear to bind in much the same position of the p-amino-benzoyl moiety of the normal substrate folic acid (7) both 3- and 4-X-analogues bind between the two red bulges above the floor. The one

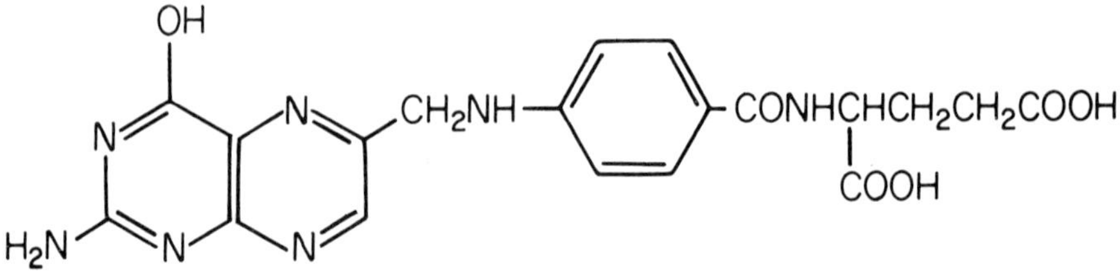

OH

H₂N, N, N, N, CH₂NH — ⟨benzene ring⟩ — CONHCHCH₂CH₂COOH, COOH (chemical structure)

7

problem with this is that such 4-X-triazines are well fitted by Eq. 10 with the low slope of 0.44 π'. If in fact they are binding like the corresponding 3-X-analogues one would expect complete desolvation with a π coefficient near 1. It is conceivable that the better binding of the 4-$CH_2ZC_6H_4$-Y group in this pocket could be exactly compensated by some steric hindrance. The solution will have to await X-ray crystallography with the inhibitor bound in place on the enzyme.

In the three case studies of QSAR and graphics based on coordinates from X-ray crystallography which we have examined there has been a general satisfying parallel between the QSAR model and the graphics model. We have not discussed the obvious aspects of such graphics. That is, from such models one can quickly understand why it would be pointless to make many kinds of derivatives. Also, as the group at the Wellcome laboratories have recently demonstrated (Kuyper *et al.*, 1982), one can design inhibitors to take advantage of special interactions with specific amino acid residues.

There is another aspect of these studies which is particularly interesting. We have felt for many years that it would be impossible to obtain good QSAR with enzymes or other bioreceptors if these receptors were not rather flexible ensembles. Our studies with the graphics and QSAR models of enzyme ligand interactions strongly support this view. For example, it is quite clear that 4-X-triazines make a bad contact with Phe-49 in *L. casei*. Nevertheless this does not prevent these inhibitors from strong binding. While the binding is less than expected the correction between observed and found log $1/K_i$ is rather well accounted for by using Charton's continuous steric parameter ν. This means there must be some "give" in positioning the inhibitors or Phe-49 or both. Actually one can see room for a small amount of movement for Phe-49. A most revealing substituent is the rigid group -C$\equiv$CC$_6$H$_5$. It is 20 times less active than Eq. 10 predicts, but it still has a log $1/K_i$ of 3.86 compared to 4.7 for the parent compound (X = H). From the crystallography as visualized in the graphics model there seems to be no way for this congener to fit without a *large* amount of give in the enzyme and/or the ligand.

It is all very well to design effective inhibitors using purified enzymes. The real question is will they be effective *in vivo*? It seems unlikely that we can understand the jump from enzyme to whole animal without some careful ground work. To this end we are studying DHFR inhibitors in cell culture (Coats *et al.*, 1981; Selassie *et al.*, 1982a,b). From these studies it is clear that DHFR may or may not be in a different state in the living cell. Some insight can be gained from a comparison of Eqs 12, 13 and 14.

Inhibition of murine leukemia (L5178Y) DHFR by 3-X-triazines (Selassie *et al.*, 1982).

$$\log 1/K_i = 1.13\,\pi' - 1.33\log(\beta.10^{\pi'} + 1) + 0.42I + 6.44 \qquad [12]$$
$$n = 38,\, r = 0.920,\, s = 0.315,\, \pi_0 = 1.44$$

Inhibition (50%) leukemia (L5178Y) cell culture sensitive to MTX (Selassie *et al.*, 1982).

$$\log 1/C = 1.32\,\pi - 1.70\log(\beta.10^{\pi} + 1) + 0.44I + 8.10 \qquad [13]$$
$$n = 37,\, r = 0.929,\, s = 0.274,\, \pi_0 = 0.76$$

Inhibition (50%) leukemia (L5178YR) cell culture resistant to MTX (Selassie *et al.*, 1982).

$$\log 1/C = 0.41\,\pi - 0.16MR + 5.24 \qquad [14]$$
$$n = 42,\, r = 0.895,\, s = 0.344$$

Equation 12 was derived from data obtained on DHFR isolated from tumour cells resistant to MTX (Eq. 14). It is not greatly different from Eq. 9 for human DHFR and it is similar to Eq. 13 for the 50% inhibition of tumour cell growth *in vitro*. This suggests that the isolated DHFR from resistant and sensitive tumour cells is much the same if not identical.

The π_0 of Eq. 13 is somewhat smaller than that for Eq. 12, probably because of sites of loss for the more lipophilic compounds to lipophilic compartments other than DHFR in the cell culture. In Eqs 13 and 14 π for all of the substituents including Y gives a better correlation than π' as one might expect since the hydrophobic character of π has a role to play in the inhibitor partitioning in and out of membranes. The more negative slope of the right hand side of the bilinear model, $(1.13-1.33 = -0.20$ vs $1.32 - 1.70 = -0.38)$ accounts for the lower activity of the highly lipophilic analogues. It was rather surprising to find the intercept of Eq. 13 1.66 log units higher than that of Eq. 12. It turns out to take about 50 times less inhibitor to achieve 50% inhibition of cell growth compared to 50% inhibition of isolated DHFR. One might have expected things to be the other way around since some of the inhibitor in the cell culture must be tied up by other macromolecules.

While Eq. 13 is much like Eq. 12, Eq. 14 is radically different. The slope with the π term is less than half that of Eqs 12 of 13. Moreover π_0 cannot be established using the bilinear model and the term in I is not present. There is a small negative term in MR which makes only a minor contribution to the SAR.

The data on which Eq. 14 is based have been fitted to a parabolic model in Eq. 15.

$$\log 1/C = 0.59\,\pi - 0.038\,\pi^2 - 0.14\,MR + 5.14 \qquad [15]$$
$$n = 42,\; r = 0.933,\; s = 0.282,\; \pi_0 = 7.7\; (6-12)$$

Even though the 95% confidence intervals are large it is clear that π_0 of Eq. 15 is much different from that of Eqs 13 or 14. In fact the small coefficient with π and the large π_0 remind one of Eq. 10 and the fit in Plate VII of the bacterial enzyme. If the DHFR in the resistant tumour cells were twisted a bit to open up the active site then long hydrophobic substituents might bind along a hydrophobic floor as in Plate VII. If such an opening of the active site did occur then the two normally observed hydrophobic bulges might be separated enough so that the special interaction of the $-CH_2ZC_6H_4-$unit would not show up. The fact that an I term does not appear in Eqs 14 or 15 tends to support this hypothesis.

Conclusion

The QSAR paradigm has been developing slowly for the past 20 years so that by now thousands of QSAR have been derived for hundreds of different systems from enzymes to whole animals. This huge amount of work shows that we are in a general way on the right tract in our efforts to unravel structure−activity relationships. No doubt many improvements and new ideas will change the scene greatly in the next decade. Despite our success, even in the minds of the "True Believer" in QSAR, there are nagging doubts about just what QSAR is telling us about any given system. Some of this doubt is being dispelled by the exploratory work which we have done with QSAR and X-ray coordinate based molecular graphics. The basic soundness of using physiochemical parameters seems justified. However, a great deal more of such work must be done with well defined purified receptors before we have anything approaching a general understanding of ligand−receptor interactions.

The next step must be study on the level of the cell because it is all too clear that receptors in the cell can react differently. Finally QSAR with the same inhibitors must be undertaken with animals. Only by laying the ground work carefully will we be able to jump quickly and with some confidence from isolated receptors to whole animals.

Many have questioned the assumption that the three-dimensional picture obtained from crystals of enzyme by X-ray studies is the same three-dimensional structure that exists in solution. We have been impressed with the good correspondence between the QSAR model derived from enzymes in solution and the graphics models based on the X-ray coordinates of the crystal. However the enzymes do show a large amount of flexibility which can best be understood from kinetic studies using substrates and inhibitors. We have been surprised at how far we have been able to go in the formulation of QSAR without excessive reliance on steric parameters or estimates of ideal conformations from quantum or molecular mechanics.

We believe the new look to QSAR provided by X-ray crystallography and molecular graphics will have a most profound affect on our understanding of the interaction of drugs with bioreceptors.

References

Baker, B.R. (1967). "Design of Active-Site Directed Irreversible Enzyme Inhibitors". Wiley, New York.

Blaney, J.M., Jorgensen, E.C., Connolly, M.L., Ferrin, T.E., Langridge, R., Gatley, S.J., Burridge, J.M. and Blake, C.C.F. (1982). *J. Med. Chem.* **25**, 785–790.

Braun, W., Bösch, C., Brown, L.R., Go, N. and Wüthrich, K. (1981). *Biochim. Biophys. Acta* **667**, 377–396.

Brown, L.R., Braun, W., Kumar, A. and Wüthrich, K. (1982). *Biophys. J.* **37**, 319–328.

Carotti, A., Smith, R.N., Wong, S., Hansch, C., Blaney, J.M. and Langridge, R. *Arch. Biochem. Biophys.*, in press.

Charton, M. (1977). *In* "Design of Biopharmaceutical Properties Through Prodrugs and Analogs" (E.B. Roche, ed.), pp. 228–281. American Pharmaceutical Association Washington, D.C.

Coates, E.A., Genther, C.S., Dietrich, S.W., Guo, Z.R. and Hansch, C. (1981). *J. Med. Chem.* **24**, 1422–1429.

Drenth, J., Jansonius, J.N., Koekoek, R., Sluyterman, L.A.A. and Wolthers, B.G. (1970). *Philos. Trans. R. Soc. London, Ser. B* **257**, 231–236.

Feldman, R.J., Bing, D.H., Furie, B.C., Furie, D. (1978). *Proc. Natl. Acad. Sci. U.S.A.* **75**, 5409–5412.

Grieco, C., Hansch, C., Silipo, C., Smith, R.N. and Vittoria, A. (1979). *Arch. Biochem. Biophys.* **194**, 542–551.

Guo, Z.R., Dietrich, S.W., Hansch, C., Dolnick, B.J. and Bertino, J.R. (1981). *Mol Pharmacol.* **20**, 649–656.

Hammett, L.P. (1970). "Physical Organic Chemistry". 2nd ed. McGraw Hill, New York.

Hansch, C. (1969). *Acc. Chem. Res.* **2**, 232–239.

Hansch, C. (1974). *J. Chem. Educ.* **51**, 360–365.

Hansch, C. and Leo, A. (1979). "Substituent Constants for Correlation Analysis in Biology and Chemistry". Wiley-Interscience.

Hansch, C., Maloney, P.P., Fujita, T. and Muir, R.M. (1962). *Nature (London)* **194**, 178–180.

Hansch, C., Grieco, C., Silipo, C. and Vittoria, A. (1977a). *J. Med. Chem.* **20**, 1420–1435.

Hansch, C., Smith, R.N., Rockoff, A., Calef, D.F., Jow, P.Y.C. and Fukunaga, J.Y. (1977b). *Arch. Biochem. Biophys.* **183**, 383–392.

Hansch, C., Li, R.L., Blaney, J.M. and Langridge, R. (1982). *J. Med. Chem.* **25**, 777–784.

Hansch, C., Hathaway, B.A., Guo, Z.R., Selassie, C.D., Dietrich, S.W., Matthews, D.A., Volz, K.W., Blaney, J.M., Langridge, R. and Kaufman, B.T. Unpublished results.

Hathaway, B.A., Guo, Z.R., Hansch, C., Delcamp, T.J., Susten, S.S. and Freisheim, J.A. Unpublished results.

Hitchings, G.H. and Smith, S.L. (1979). *Adv. Enzyme. Regul.* **18**, 349–371.

Ingold, C.K. (1969). "Structure and Mechanism in Organic Chemistry". 2nd ed. Cornell University Press, Ithaca, N.Y.

Kubinyi, H. and Kehrhahn, O.H. (1978). *Arznei-Forsch.* **28**, 598–601.

Kuyper, L.F., Roth, B., Baccanari, D.P., Ferone, D., Beddell, C.R., Champness, J.N., Stammers, D.K., Dann, J.G., Norrington, F.E.A., Baker, D.J. and Goodford, P.J. (1982). *J. Med. Chem.* **25**, 1120–1122.

Langridge, R., Ferrin, T.E., Kuntz, I.D. and Connolly, M.L. (1981). *Science* **211**, 661–666.

Li, R.L., Hansch, C., Matthews, D., Blaney, J.M., Langridge, R., Delcamp, T.J., Susten, S.S. and Freisheim, J.H. (1982). *Quant. Struct. Act. Rel.* **1**, 1–7.

Matthews, D.A., Alden, R.A., Bolin, J.T., Filman, D.J., Freer, S.T., Hamlin, R., Hol, W.G.J., Kisliuk, R.L., Pastore, E.J., Plante, L.T., Suong, N. and Kraut, J. (1978). *J. Biol. Chem.* **253**, 6946–6954.

Matthews, D.A., Alden, R.A., Freer, S.T., Xuong, N.H. and Kraut, J. (1979). *J. Biol. Chem.* **254**, 4144–4151.

Partington, J.R. (1935). "Origins and Development of Applied Chemistry", p. 185. Longmans Green and Company, London.

Quigley, G.J., Wang, A.H.J., Ughetto, G., van der Marvel, G., van Boom, J.H. and Rich, A. (1980). *Proc. Natl. Acad. Sci. U.S.A.* **77**, 7204–7208.

Selassie, C.D., Guo, Z.R., Hansch, C., Khwaja, T.A. and Pentecost, S. (1982a). *J. Med. Chem.* **25**, 518–522.

Selassie, C.D., Li, R.L., Hansch, C., Khwaja, T.A. and Dias, C.B. (1982b). *J. Med. Chem.* **25**, 157–161.

Silipo, C., Hansch, C., Grieco, C. and Vittoria, A. (1979). *Arch. Biochem. Biophys.* **194**, 552–557.

Smith, R.N., Hansch, C., Kim, K.H., Omiya, B., Fukumura, G., Selassie, C.D., Jow, P.Y.C., Blaney, J.M. and Langridge, R. (1982) *Arch. Biochem. Biophys.* **215**, 319–328.

Taft, R.W. Jr. (1956). *In* "Steric Effects in Organic Chemistry" (M.S. Newman, ed.), Ch. 13. John Wiley, New York.

Tsai, S.C., Tsa, C.C. and Sobell, H.M. (1977). *J. Mol. Biol.* **114**, 301–331.

Unger, S.H. (1980). *In* "Drug Design" vol. IX (E.J. Ariens, ed.), 48–115. Academic Press, New York.

Volz, K.W., Matthews, D.A., Alden, R.A., Freer, S.T., Hansch, C., Kaufman, B.T. and Kraut, J. (1982). *J. Biol. Chem.* **257**, 2528–2536.

Discussion

Chairman: Professor Whalley

Professor Whalley

First, I would like to suggest that Professor Hansch's contribution has been a eutectic point, or a nexus. It has been a really key point so far in the whole presentation, and I suspect that it may remain so. He has shown very elegantly, and in his own words has stated quite clearly, one concept which was repeatedly referred to previously in less definitive terms — namely, that at least some enzyme surfaces are not particularly rigid.

My second point concerns a question of semantics in this symposium so far which has not really been addressed — but it is not totally a question of semantics. "Drug design: fact or fantasy?" is open to numerous interpretations. We have been presented with one interpretation very eloquently and elegantly by all the previous contributors — namely, having got an active compound, how to get it more appropriately to the site, how, by modification in transport and so on, it can perhaps be made more active than it would be (because it can be delivered more appropriately to where it should act). But, of course, before we can get an active compound to a site, we have to catch an active compound. I think that it is not without significance that 75% plus of Professor Hansch's contribution was concerned with what is probably the largest family of compounds which was devised relatively simplistically (I say that with great respect to the people who did it) on the basis of a theory which held up. It produced trimethoprim, methotrexate, allopurinol and, more recently, acyclovir.

This is the other aspect of the problem which we have to address, and which I hope we will address, in the remainder of this conference: how we zero in, as it were, on the seminal compounds which will be capable of modification, which can be looked at in the elegant way in which Professor Hansch has looked at his compounds. He has amply demonstrated how, probably fortuitously, but none the less realistically, the substances which were derived such a long time back ideally fit into these clefts, into these cavities, into these spaces. He has so eloquently and graphically (literally as well as metaphorically) illustrated the manner in which these compounds actually work in the dihydrofolate reductive enzyme system.

When we come to the syndicate discussions, I suggest that this may very well be one of the points that we would wish to discuss rather more extensively.

Professor Stevens
The classical inhibitors of this enzyme, dihydrofolate reductase, have all been concerned with mimicking structural features of the substrate — that is, dihydrofolate. What about the forgotten interactions between the co-factor and the enzyme? Is there not scope for the design of a whole new series of inhibitors of this enzyme, which mimic the binding of the co-factor? Is there any progress along those lines?

Professor Hansch
Yes, I think there is — there is good potential there. There are a couple of things that would worry me about embarking on that: first, the chemistry. Those molecules have fairly complicated chemistry, but it might be possible to simplify the chemistry, and to make part of it in a simpler way. That is fairly formidable.

Secondly, there are a lot of other enzymes in the living systems that use NADPH. If their receptors turn out to be somewhat like this receptor, we might get into trouble there. I feel, though, that the substrate part of the receptor is very likely to be unique. The other part may also be unique — I do not know, but there will be problems if many molecules turn out to have much the same receptor.

I showed how I would try to get a double inhibitor, and what we are going to try to do. That is, to push something in there far enough, and anchor it firmly enough so as to keep the NADPH off. I do not know whether it will be possible to do that, but we will try it.

Professor Marshall

The crystal-bound structure of NAD has been solved in perhaps four, five or six cases now. It binds in an extremely similar way. It is almost possible to lay those things on top of each other in five or six enzymes. I would expect, therefore, that NADP would probably turn out to be analogous.

I am curious about the actual mechanics of putting the models in, about the energy. Was any sort of feedback being used, in terms of rough energies or anything? Was this all done manually?

Professor Hansch

It was all taken from the tapes. We got the tapes from Kraut and Matthews or Brookhaven and just put those things on. In some cases, we have tried to move things a little. But, at this point, we have not felt it necessary to take any liberty with the structure — because everything fits beautifully. We have now run over 100 of these triazines and about 50 benzylpyrimidines, and we find quite a good correspondence between what we got with the QSAR and what we put in. What that means to me is that what the crystallographer is telling us is quite near to what it is.

What the crystallographer is not telling us — and he cannot do so very well — is the flexibility. I would like to illustrate this, to show how that can be quite upsetting.

A post-doctorial assistant (Bruce Hathaway) made a compound. I thought it was a bad idea, but let him go ahead with it. I was right — partly. He liked acetylene chemistry, so he thought it would be fun to make that derivative. From what we already knew, I thought that it would not be a very effective inhibitor. It turned out to be a bad inhibitor on isolated dihydrofolate reductases of all kinds.

We started testing this compound on tumour cells — on two kinds, those sensitive to methotrexate and those resistant to methotrexate. In the sensitive cells it is a very bad fit by QSAR — it is off by two orders of magnitude. But on the resistant cells it is a perfect fit, with no problem at all.

If we look at the graphics, it is clear why it is a bad fit on the sensitive dihydrofolate reductase — it looks as though on the dihydrofolate reductase it has to cut a phenylalanine in half on binding. It has to go right through a phenylalanine.

What is fascinating about it is that although it is bad from our point of view — it misses by two orders of magnitude — it still binds quite tightly. I do not think that it is cutting phenylalanine in half. That means, therefore, that perhaps the rest of it can "give" in its binding, or the enzyme, or something, "gives" − because there are all kinds of "give" in that system which would not have been anticipated from the crystallography, or from the QSAR either. It was not seen until we started testing it on the resistant cells.

I could give other examples. There are lots of things that we have seen, many small examples, showing that these enzymes are really very complex microcosms, and that there is a lot of movement within them which is still not understood, or can be explained or really be anticipated.

Professor Roques

It seems to me that in this country, at Cambridge, Jim Feeney and J.C.K. Roberts have shown by NMR spectroscopy that methotrexate analogues are able to change their conformation within the active site of the enzyme. Did Professor Hansch check the possibility of a change in conformational states of the analogue within the active site, exhibiting a very great degree of freedom within the active site of the enzyme, dihydrofolate reductase?

Professor Hansch

I showed that first example, when we were comparing how methotrexate bound and how folic acid bound. Feeney and Roberts contributed to the understanding of that problem. But when we are looking at this, playing around with the molecules, there are many different ways in which these substrates can be bound. All the possibilities will not be known until a great deal of crystallography has been done.

In the case of papain which I showed, and which I thought was a good example, we fell into a trap. Everything fitted perfectly, we made the next series, we thought we understood, and then we discovered that we did not understand it. If some minimization studies had been done, calculating whether it would be one way or another, I do not think it would have been possible to make any predictions about which way they would bind. The only way it can be done is the way that the medicinal chemists always do it − make the molecules and test them to see what happens.

Dr Bost

Could Professor Hansch's representation be useful in terms of designing transition state analogues?

Professor Hansch

Yes, I think it would be useful. I am not too excited about transition state analogues because (as was discussed previously) I do not know when we have one and when we do not. There can be something that looks like a transition state analogue (as Professor Andrews said), and variations on it can be made. I do not really think much in those terms − but with any kind of inhibitors, graphics are an enormous help. We can see when there is a hydrophobic surface against which to work. In all three cases in which we have looked for interaction, and there has been a hydrophobic surface indicated from the QSAR, we have found it when we have looked at the enzyme. So I think that what has been known intuitively for a long term is really there.

11 The Virtues of Present Strategies for Drug Discovery

K.R.H. WOOLDRIDGE

May and Baker Ltd.,
Dagenham, Essex RM10 7XS, Great Britain

Introduction

The main theme of the Round Table Conference is to question whether Drug Design is Fact or Fantasy at the present time. Most of the participants are experts in various specialist fields and as a contrast the present contribution is intended to take a broad view of drug discovery as seen from the viewpoint of a Research Manager of an innovative pharmaceutical company.

It may be argued that the drug industry has ben successful in introducing a wide variety of effective new drugs during the last 30–40 years. To achieve this position various strategies have been followed, and it is important to know why these approaches were adopted, to examine how cost-effective they are, and to ask whether they are still relevant today, and if not to what extent they could or should be replaced by newer approaches.

The Evolution of a New Medical Product

The various stages of the evolution of a new medical product are indicated in Fig. 1. A clear understanding of the objectives of the research project must be reached and it is crucial to appreciate that these objectives are clinical conditions or disease processes. The scientists involved

DRUG DESIGN: FACT OR FANTASY
ISBN 0.12.388180.3

Evolution of a new medical product

Set Objectives		
Devise Research Strategy		
Establish Suitable Test Procedures		3–10 years
Obtain and Evaluate Test Compounds		
Select Potential Product		
Toxicology	Process Development	
Formulation	Production	
Clinical Trials	Patents	7 years
Registration	etc.	
Marketing		

FIG. 1

in drug research have to translate medical objectives into a set of problems or subsidiary objectives which are capable of being solved in the laboratory. Not the least of these problems is to establish a suitable laboratory test or tests which are predictive for the target disease process. This is the first problem for the biologist or biochemist and only when meaningful evaluation techniques are available can the task of looking for potential products begin. The next problems involve obtaining or selecting test compounds, evaluating them, and hopefully choosing a candidate product. The time-scale for this phase of the operation is open-ended depending on the magnitude of the clinical problem and the willingness of the company to continue financing the project.

Once selected on the basis of laboratory tests there is still at the best a seven to eight year period of development which, if all goes smoothly, will lead to the marketing of the new product.

Feeding the Biological Screen

When suitable tests have been established which are believed to be predictive for the human disease process, the problem resolves into the question of feeding the biological screen. Figure 2 illustrates how traditionally the pharmaceutical industry has approached this problem and the following sections describe some of the advantages and disadvantages of each approach.

Modification of Active Compounds by Specific Chemical Synthesis

Using an active molecule as a starting point has obvious attractions. It is highly motivating for the synthetic organic chemist because he will

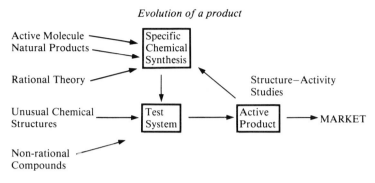

FIG. 2

almost certainly make active new molecules. It is feasible to employ sophisticated evaluation techniques because the number of new compounds will be relatively low. Often it is possible to define precisely the biological properties required e.g. to retain a certain level of activity but to have a lower specific side-effect.

A major disadvantage is that any product obtained is likely to have only marginal advantages over its predecessors, the so-called "me too" product. With the high cost of development such a product may be unattractive commercially. This could be unfortunate in the long term because successive minor improvements in a family of drugs may lead to a very substantial improvement overall. Another possible disadvantage is that because competitors may also base their chemistry on the same active molecule they may follow similar paths leading to duplication and possible patent conflicts.

This approach gives full rein to the ingenuity of the organic chemist who is able to change rings, interchange functional groups, make isosteres, or perhaps incorporate the amidine skeleton into a bewildering variety of structures.

However, the great advantage of this approach is that it obviously leads to new drugs. A recent book (Bindra and Lednicer, 1982) lists 12 examples of drugs marketed in the last few years and a high proportion of them appear to have resulted from chemical modification of an earlier drug or active product.

Rational Theory

If something is known about the biochemistry and pharmacology of the disease process, it may be possible to exert a beneficial effect by modifying a particular metabolic pathway. If an enzymatic process is involved, the natural substrate or known inhibitors may provide starting points. It may also be possible to use *in vitro* assay techniques avoiding the use of live animals in the preliminary screen, and reducing costs.

The disadvantage is that the enzyme reaction or pharmacological receptor may be yet a further stage removed from the prime objective which is the disease process in man. This could give rise to such problems as modifying molecules which may have the required properties in an isolated enzyme system or a receptor-rich isolated tissue so that they retain the activity *in vivo*. Another possible problem may arise if the biochemical or pharmacological rationale may not be a complete reflection of the disease process.

However this approach has been successful historically, for example in the fields of folate antagonists and H_2 receptor antagonists.

Non-Rational or Random Screening

The method of screening large numbers of compounds or microbial products from any available source in a battery of tests is the approach which is most often associated with the pharmaceutical industry and is often bitterly attacked. Most certainly it has many disadvantages; it requires extensive and often expensive tests and it may be demotivating to the scientists unless they are trying to develop new tests or are motivated by their involvement in an important problem. Otherwise intellectual input is very low. Perhaps the biggest disadvantage is that the time scale is unpredictable because a lead may emerge after a short period of screening or on the other hand nothing may be found after examining hundreds of thousands of compounds over many years.

However, his approach has been successful historically, for example table activity in chemical series which may lead to whole new families of drugs. In the case of microbial products it evaluates complex chemical structures which it is highly unlikely would be arrived at by a rational theory or by chance synthesis.

The great attraction of this technique is in areas where there are no active molecules and not enough is known of the pharmacology or biochemistry to suggest a rational approach. Alternatively, even when there are active molecules and mechanistic knowledge, it may be a requirement for a product operating by a new mechanism to overcome resistance or adaptation.

Unusual Chemistry

This approach involves the speculative synthesis of unusual structures and testing very widely to pick up any biological activity. It enables the chemist to be highly innovative in his own field but the chances of success are low. In many eyes this approach is a variation of random screening with the added cost of synthesing the speculative molecules.

Why Drug Design is Necessary

The cost of finding, developing and marketing a new drug substance taking into account the cost of unsuccessful research and development work has been put as high as £89 million in 1981 (Dench, 1981). Of this figure the synthesis and screening of test compounds was estimated at £26 million assuming a success rate of 1 in 10 000. It is clear that this enormous figure may be regarded as a target which could be reduced by effective drug design. Any technique which can be shown to improve the chance of success and reduce the number of compounds that need to be synthesized or extracted and screened will appear attractive unless of course the gains are eroded because of the cost of the new approach. This reasoning applies to techniques which allow rapid optimization of a lead compound but could be particularly valuable if the techniques enabled new leads to be generated.

The Place of Drug Design

If it is accepted that drug design is possible it is constructive to consider the circumstances where it could reduce costs. Figure 3 gives a generalized picture of the research strategy which can be adopted taking into account the state of knowledge of the disease problem.

When a great deal is known about the biochemistry and pharmacology of the disease process, drug design may well fill a place.

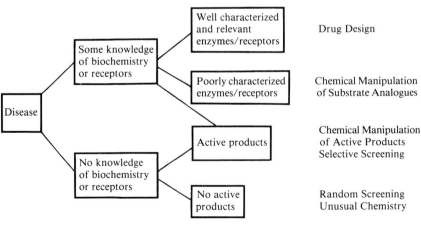

FIG. 3

Unfortunately many of the major problems such as atherosclerosis or arthritis, fall into areas where not enough is known of the biochemical mechanisms to enable a rational approach to be contemplated.

It may be argued that in such cases, research resources should be devoted to basic research in order to achieve a better understanding of the problem. However this is a long term solution and if a shorter term answer is required there has been no alternative to resorting to random screening or the modification of active products if known. There is a great need for a technique which could use the information inherent in active structures, or inactive structures, to design new molecules with the required activity. It may be that pattern recognition is such a technique.

There is no doubt that once a good lead has been uncovered, application of QSAR techniques should minimize the time and resources required to optimize the series. Suitably designed analogues spanning ranges of partition, steric, and electronic parameters should enable a model to be deduced which will enable rapid optimization (Wooldridge, 1980).

Pitfalls in Drug Design

In the previous sections, an attempt has been made to discuss where drug design could fit into the broad strategy of drug discovery used historically by industry. To complete the picture, some of the possible pitfalls in drug design should be considered.

The worst situation is that traditional approaches are reduced to finance a specialist group of drug designers who then head in a direction unlikely to produce useful products. This is an extreme view but there are many pitfalls which it may be useful to enumerate.

Poor or Remote Data

Drug design is often very dependent on the availability of good data to suggest a theory, mechanism or model, and it is crucial that the facts on which the approach is based are correct. This is an obvious problem but unfortunately easily overlooked. One of the factors is that biological scientists and physical scientists often have very different viewpoints. For example the chemist can define his compounds precisely whereas the biologist needs to generalize the limits where the change in a biological system can be reproduced reliably. Biologists tend to distrust *in vitro* biological data as being too remote from the clinical situation whereas the chemists like them because they give reproducible figures.

These differences are fundamental but are minimized when the biologist and chemist or physicist or mathematician work together. The danger is that the drug designer may work in isolation without the restraining or realistic influence of a biologist.

The Wrong Mechanism of Action

This is the rather obvious possibility that a rational approach based on a biochemical model of the disease process may founder because of an imperfect understanding of the mechanism. It is quite possible to produce a very effective enzyme inhibitor only to find that additional properties are necessary for an effective drug and that the hard-won inhibitor does not work.

Outliers

The problem of outliers, poles, quantum leaps etc. is particularly worrying when attempting to optimize a lead in a chemical family. A small change in structure may increase (or decrease) activity a great deal more than predicted by the mathematical model. This effect may be accommodated by the use of dummy variables to ensure conformity with the model but usually the structural feature causing the change is unpredictable. The scientist with an active series may devise a mathematical model and use this to optimize the series to give "the best compound", but is left with the problem of coping with the quantum leap. Is the only answer to make many structural variations in the hope of achieving an unexpected jump in activity. Is not this in fact the traditional approach?

Elimination of Intelligence

Advanced technology is usually but not always associated with computers and complex programs. This has its dangers and by way of illustration it may be worth considering some of the laws and maxims enshrined in the literature.

Gallois's revelation

If you put rubbish into a computer, nothing comes out but rubbish. But this rubbish having passed through an expensive machine is somehow ennobled, and no-one dares to criticize it (Dickson, 1980).

Gall's law

Any large system is going to be operating most of the time in failure mode (Gall, 1978).

Computer maxim
To err is human but to really foul things up requires a computer (Dickson, 1980).

The great danger is that the scientist may come to depend on, or even worship, the computer and his thought processes may become channelled or inhibited. Very many effective drugs have been discovered by serendipity and it is essential for the scientist to be aware of what is happening in related fields and to think laterally and constructively. This viewpoint has given rise to perhaps what may be a more realistic maxim.

Wooldridge's law
Make the blighters think!

Conclusion

In this paper, an attempt has been made to put the newer approaches to drug design into context and to look realistically at the potential and the pitfalls. Most certainly new approaches have their place and will have an increasing influence on research strategy. However it must be stressed that the real objective of drug research is to cure diseases afflicting mankind, and the new approaches will have to prove their worth in competition with the traditional, and not unsuccessful, methods of attacking the prime problems.

References

Bindra, I.S. and Lednicer, D. (1982). "Chronicles of Drug Discovery". John Wiley, New York.
Dench, W. (1981). A.B.P.I.* News, No. 185, 5.
Dickson, P. (1980). "The Official Rules". Arrow Books, London.
Gall, J. (1978). "Systemantics: How Systems Work and Especially How They Fail". Wildwood House, London.
Wooldridge, K.R.H. (1980). *Eur. J. Med. Chem.–Chim. Ther.* **15**, 63–66.

* Association of the British Pharmaceutical Industry.

12 Traditional or Pragmatic Research

M. MESSER

*Directeur des Recherches Chimiques et Biochimiques
Pharmaceutiques, Rhône-Poulenc Recherches, Centre
Nicolas Grillet, B.P. 14 F 94400 Vitry-sur-Seine, France*

Introduction

The history of the pharmaceutical industry shows that most major drugs were discovered by a combination of opportunity and luck. These days it is unreasonable to expect that this approach will continue to be the most productive and it is preferable to employ a more rational approach.

The traditional approaches to drug research in the industry have been subjected to criticism directed particularly at the medicinal chemist who is accused of carrying out interesting chemistry, the products of which are screened blindly for biological activity. This is far from reality and in fact the development of molecular pharmacology and advances in physical chemistry, biochemistry and biology have resulted in considerable harmony between chemists and biologists over structure – activity relationships.

The Objectives

Those involved in therapeutic research usually have in mind the objective of discovering a drug which will provide a genuine advance in a given pharmaceutical field.

A patient will consider a drug as an improvement if it will allow him

DRUG DESIGN: FACT OR FANTASY
ISBN 0.12.388180.3

Copyright © 1984 by Academic Press London.
All rights of reproduction in any form reserved.

to recover faster with fewer side-effects. This may be achieved in a number of ways, for example higher potency leading to reduced dosage, modification of the pharmacokinetic profile to improve the therapeutic effect, or a more acceptable route of administration.

Another improvement may consist of a wider range of activity leading to an enlarged field of application. Toxicity and side-effects due to the biotransformation of the drug to toxic metabolites may be reduced in an analogue even if the potency is not improved.

However, the greatest advance that can be achieved is when a new drug attacks the root cause of the disease process. Many drugs alleviate the symptoms but do not provide a cure. A compound, whatever its level of activity, which is curative represents real innovation.

Scientific Requirements and Industrial Restraints

The development of a new drug in industry must take into account the difference in the quality of the compound as perceived by the physician today and how it will be perceived in ten years time when competition and progress in fundamental research may totally change the situation. Industrial realism requires innovation not for itself but as a safety margin for the future and this is one of its most important features.

TABLE 1

	A	B	C	D
Chemical novelty	0	+	0	+
Biological novelty	0	0	+	+
Innovation	0	+	+ +	+ + +

In fact, we may imagine four different situations as can be seen in Table 1 where the innovative level of a drug is related to its chemical novelty as well as to the novelty or type of biological test leading to its discovery.

In situation A with little or no chemical or biological novelty, there is no innovation. In the situation B where there is chemical novelty but no biological improvement, innovation is marginal but it may raise the fundamental question of why structurally different classes of drug can produce the same biological response. Situation C represents the case of the discovery of new biological properties of known drugs and may be regarded as a major scientific advance. Further work may well lead to more active and perhaps specific drugs. Of course in the final situation D, novel chemistry and biology is truly a rare dish providing kudos from the scientific community and laying a foundation for future advances in therapy.

Drug Research Strategies

The discovery of a new drug may stem from one of the following strategies.

1) The improvement of the potency of known active compounds by chemical modification.
2) The design of compounds on a rational biological hypothesis.
3) The synthesis of novel chemical molecules with a "biological look".

Each of these possible approaches will be discussed in depth from the point of view of their innovative efficiency.

The Improvement of the Potency of Known Active Compounds by Chemical Modification

This approach, to make something new from something old, is usually followed when the established biological properties are basically satisfactory, and furthermore, there are no more original ideas to pursue.

This strategy does present psychological advantages in that everybody gets something out of it, the chemist will make active compounds and the biologists and toxicologists will have the opportunity to make comparisons with reference compounds.

A good optimization starts from an active compound as a lead and produces a new compound with a better ratio between relevant parameters such as potency, side-effects, duration of action, cost etc.

In order to make best use of the research team, the medicinal chemist tries to consider the following questions.

1) What are the relevant chemical or physicochemical parameters?
2) Which parts of the molecule are important and may be modified sterically, electronically or have their lipophilic character changed?
3) How may the biological properties be modified?

To answer these questions the medicinal chemist may have to take into account many physicochemical properties such as electronic distribution, lipophilicity, and molecular geometry. Van der Waals radii, pK values, molecular refraction indexes, spectroscopic properties, and other parameters may have to be determined. Also he may make use of molecular orbital calculations and a variety of statistical techniques.

Suitable use of these parameters should in theory help the chemist to identify and select from many possible chemical structures those variants which may lead to the optimum effect. If rational optimization is to be worthwhile therapeutically and commercially, the product should be a molecule with a novel chemical structure.

In order to assess the results of optimization, approximately 30 drugs, either already marketed or in late development, were considered. All these products were presumably selected after optimization of the parent chemical series, in some cases at least, by the application of sophisticated QSAR techniques. However, the survey revealed a consistent pattern: the selected compounds are often "outliers"; the most effective aromatic substituents are Cl, F, CH_3O, CH_3 or sometimes CF_3; the selected compound is usually amongst the 20 or 30 which are the most obvious and easy to synthesize; the other compounds in the series (usually 100 to 200) are synthesized in order to provide good patent cover.

It may be concluded that although it is often claimed that a large variety of compounds needs to be studied to select the optimum one, in practice a reasonable optimization may be achieved from a few compounds. Within the limits of a chemical series, optimization is fairly routine.

Therefore using existing drugs as a starting point and hoping still to achieve innovation is a hazardous strategy because optimization may well have been achieved already.

The Design of Compounds on a Rational Biological Hypothesis

To base the design of a compound on a rational hypothesis, the chemist needs to consider several points.

1) The mechanism of action of a given compound.
2) The possibility that different chemical series may act by the same biological mechanism.
3) Whether enough information is available at the molecular level to design active compounds.

Mechanism of action

Biological activity may be rationalized if it stems from the chemical or physicochemical properties of the series. For example the alkylating properties of compounds such as the nitrogen mustards, the nitrosoureas and the mitomycins, or the cross-linking properties of *cis*-platinum derivatives relate to their anti-cancer activity. The activity of anthracyclines, ellipticine, and the anthracene diones has been shown to be due to intercalation in the double helix of DNA. The anti-coccidial polyether ionophores are potent complexing agents for mono- and divalent cations.

The biological action of a compound is also readily explicable if it mimics a natural substrate or mediator. This is the case with suicide substrates, antimetabolites, for the angiotensin converting enzyme inhibitors, and for analogues of mediators such as PAF, GABA, and enkephalins.

However in many cases the mechanism of the biological activity is unknown because the target activity has not yet been clearly identified. This is the case with benzodiazepines and other psychotropic series, the non-steroidal anti-inflammatories and antisecretory agents.

Different chemical series acting by the same biochemical mechanism

Psychotropics   Members of quite different chemical series appear to act on the same pharmacological receptors e.g. diazepam and suriclone (R.P. 31264).

Suriclone   Diazepam

The activity of the parent chemical series was discovered by serendipity and it is disturbing that there are no rational structural similarities. It may be that the application of more sophisticated techniques may reveal some structural analogies but for the moment the only consolation is that the receptor may not be particularly specific or that there may be other relevant factors, which leaves ample scope for future developments.

Antisecretory agents   The H_2-receptor antagonist story shows a progression from burinamide through metiamide and cimetidine to ranitidine.

Burimamide was synthesized on a rational basis, and further modification led to cimetidine in which the introduction of the cyanoamide

Burimamide (1970)
(SKF)

Metiamide (1971)
(SKF)

Cimetidine (1972)
(SKF)

Ranitidine (1976)
(Glaxo)

function represented an innovative chemical change. The imidazole ring was regarded by the SKF chemists as essential, so it is surprising that ranitidine not only contains a furan nucleus but also a different side-chain. For those interested in drug design it poses the question as to what the structural analogies are between cimetidine and ranitidine. Admittedly both contain the chain $-CH_2CH_2CH_2NHCXNH-$ but this group was not conceived as fundamental in the thinking which led to burimamide. Could it be that these products arose from serendipity rather than from a logical design?

Availability of information

In theory, it should be possible to design a drug via the following steps.

1) A thorough investigation of the aetiology of the disease process.
2) The identification of the relevant pathological stages.
3) The isolation of the appropriate receptor, enzyme, or mediator.
4) The determination of chemical structure of the receptor, enzyme, or mediator.
5) Design and synthesis of the drug.

Unfortunately this sequence involves in many cases a great deal of fundamental work and it is not always possible to wait until this is done. In practice, assumptions may have to be made about the biochemical mechanisms involved in order to provide a target for the chemist. Alternatively, one may reasonably expect to find promising new compounds by starting from known active products. In this case drug design may be directed towards the synthesis of prodrugs, precursors, or more potent products using optimization procedures.

The Synthesis of Novel Chemical Molecules with a "Biological Look"

It is a general and well-accepted policy to search for products from natural sources such as plants, marine organisms etc., and to study their biological properties. Certainly some natural products such as tetrodoxin, histrionicotoxin and veratridin have remarkable properties and it may well be that other natural products with a high affinity for receptors may be found.

However during the last few years much progress has been made in the fields of receptorology, mediating agents and enzymatic interactions. A much more attractive approach is to synthesize chemically interesting molecules with a "biological look" provided that it is kept in mind that the objective is to generate a new lead. It has to be appreciated that pharmaceutical companies throughout the world synthesize some 60,000 compounds per year and this enormous competition requires the chemist to be realistic, efficient, innovative and above all to be critically selective. The necessary thought processes involve hypothesis and analysis leading to the selection of a chemical series which it is hoped will have the required biological activity.

Hypothesis
Biological macromolecules such as proteins, enzymes and cell walls have a general affinity for certain chemical groups or substructures.

1) Chemical groups or combinations of groups and heteroatoms may form a structural configuration which could show non-specific affinity for biomacromolecules due to hydrogen bonding, the formation of charge transfer complexes or transition states with low energy levels.
2) The presence of such a configuration in a molecular framework provides a pharmacophore conferring biological activity in the series. By modifying physicochemical parameters, degrees of freedom etc. it may then be possible for example to change non-specific affinity into specific affinity for a receptor.
3) Modifications of the molecular framework may generate new pharmacophores so that the nature of the affinity is modified giving rise to other types of biological activity.

Analysis
The chemical structure of a molecule possessing biological activity of any type should be studied with a view to identifying the pharmacophore. The relative influence of the pharmacophore and the general molecular framework on the overall physicochemical parameters of the molecule should also be assessed.

Selection

The selection of molecules to be synthesized is not a random chemical approach feeding blind biological screens. The chemical approach is based on experience and knowledge of the literature to suggest new substructures, new molecular frameworks or new combinations of substructures and frameworks.

Conclusion

For us, there is no doubt that, presently, synthesizing new molecules with a "biological look" has, in many cases, the highest potential for discovering new leads; even if serendipity is still involved in this strategy, it also enables an immediate use of any available theoretical information.

We know that there are causative relationships between drug structure and biological activity and that techniques are emerging which will enable us to understand these relationships better. The medicinal chemist will explore any method which will give him a better understanding of the properties of the molecules he makes and help him to predict with greater accuracy the properties of hypothetical molecules.

Today, we try to make the best of present scientific knowledge; as new methods become available progressively, we shall of course be happy to call on them in order to estimate their versatility and limitations.

13 General Discussion of Session II

CHAIRMAN: PROFESSOR WHALLEY

Professor Whalley

The fact that we are considering the question as to how drug design may be achieved indicates quite clearly that drug design will continue. It also indicates that our hosts, as one of the major pharmaceutical companies in the world, propose to remain in the business of drug design.

This brings us up against a problem which has enormous influence upon us all, no matter what our interest may be in the scientific question of how we obtain biologically active compounds. It is increasingly costly, and demands increasing resources, to pursue the type of investigations which are the subject of our discussions at this meeting. To put it more succinctly, as in so many other aspects of science, as a general statement, the minimum critical mass of an effective group gets larger.

It is also clear, I believe, that if we investigate just one chosen area, with the major objective of producing a new therapeutic agent, it is well known that the chances of success are relatively low. Therefore, as the saying goes, in order to hedge our bets, we have to be in, say, three, four or fives areas at a time.

As a consequence of this, and it may be seen throughout the world, the true innovators, the survivors who are to be innovators in this sense of producing new therapeutic agents, are inexorably being reduced in number.

Additionally, there is the problem that because of the increasing cost more and more objectives become less attractive. Unless we have a new form of therapy which is sufficiently significant, and which is sufficiently widely applicable, clearly there is no point in undertaking the research to produce it because we shall not break even. Since we must at least break even in order to stay in business, realistically we do not start.

Clearly, in the light of these considerations, the ability, by whatever process or combination of processes, to devise an appropriate strategy for the production of new therapeutic agents is absolutely vital to the survival of the pharmaceutical industry internationally as we now know it.

In a sense we have reached a parting of the ways, in that it would appear that all the victories which were capable of easy achievement have been achieved. It is clear from what has been said so far at this meeting, and in other places at other times, that in order to move forward now, a concerted attack is needed, on many of the biological processes which are very ill-understood, which are involved in many disease states. I have a suspicion that substantially the only people who can and will do this effectively are the people in the pharmaceutical industry. From now on, therefore, they must be even more committed to research – and to fundamental research – as a necessary adjunct to producing what might be called "mission-orientated" research.

If those submissions are accepted, perhaps we might look at the views which have been presented to us by Professor Wooldridge and Dr Messer acting, under instructions, as Devil's advocates.

Dr Messer indicated that we ought to make new compounds and that there was no point in looking at old compounds. As a relatively old-fashioned chemist (and I can cite some examples in support of my thesis), I still think that there must be many old compounds with novel activities that have never been observed. I say this for a whole variety of reasons. I am sure that my friend and colleague, Professor Ollis, recalls how he and I, as old "oxygen heterocycle men", for many years were not able to interest anybody in oxygen heterocycles being biologically active. It was also said that they could not be biologically active because they contained no nitrogen. But Intal was not very far removed, and many similar compounds are only "carboxyxanthones", many of which category have been known for long periods of time.

Such a very simple compound as 7-methoxy-2,2-dimethyl-δ_3-chromene, which has been known for 40 or 50 years as a natural product, a trivial compound by any standards, is now recognized as having tremendous significance in certain areas of insect biochemistry – and so it goes on. I believe that we ought to look at new compounds, but I am sure that there is a lot of mileage in many old compounds – provided that we know where to start.

Professor Wooldridge
May I add, in connection with looking at old compounds, does Professor Whalley feel sufficiently strongly that these compounds should be synthesized at the cost say of £1200 each?

Professor Whalley
No, I do not – but what I am really saying is that one's mind should not be closed to the fact that in other circumstances old compounds may be re-isolated in a different context, and be shown to have an activity which hitherto was wholly unsuspected. That might provide the incentive to go back to look (as Dr Messer has indicated) at associated compounds, analogues, homologues and so on – which is a normal process.

Professor Roques
I believe that nowadays one cannot deal with drug design without a close collaboration between chemists or biochemists and biologists. Perhaps this can be illustrated by a point I picked up in Dr Messer's talk concerning

tranquillizers, namely, how to find analogies between two families of drugs which achieve the same activity. However, dealing with tranquillizers means sophisticated mechanisms and so before discussion one must check if these compounds interact with the same receptors in a competitive or non-competitive manner and this cannot be achieved without a close collaboration with biologists involved in receptorology.

Dr Messer

I am quite happy that Professor Roques was slightly shocked by my talk. It was my purpose to provoke everyone in this meeting by giving some real facts, however annoying they may be because they underline the requirements of industrial drug design. Truly, the only worthwhile work is that which allows us to reach the final goal. There is not always a fit between *in vitro* biochemical requirements and *in vivo* efficiency. It is one of the drawbacks of rational drug design.

Dr Julou

Concerning the comparison between suriclone and diazepam and more generally between the cyclopyrrolone and benzodiazepine families, the biological studies show that the cyclopyrrolones fit very well in the classical set of tests which allow the determination of the benzodiazepine profile. Furthermore at the receptor level the same analogy was found: benzodiazepines can wipe out cyclopyrrolones from their receptors and the reverse is also true.

Professor Wermuth

I was surprised by Dr Messer's arguments. From his talk it appears that fantasy has not a large place in industrial drug research because the goal is to put a drug on the market. But the approaches he emphasized give a large place to imagination and creativity. Would it not be wiser to start with the therapeutic requirements?

Dr Messer

At the beginning, there is imagination and creativity, stemming from our knowledge and from published results either in literature or patents. But there is also a deep reflection on chemical possibilities with regard to our industrial capacities and also an attempt to estimate the biological potential of the forthcoming series on the basis of our biological knowledge and with respect to the company's therapeutic aims.

Professor Wermuth

But anyway would it not be better to start with these therapeutic aims?

Dr Messer

The therapeutic aims are carefully assessed. But I am still waiting for someone who can tell us what kind of structure, worth marketing in ten years, should be synthesized. Of course I hope this will happen, thanks to the tools the potency of which you are improving. At the present time there are only two companies which are well off for tranquillizers: Hoffmann-La Roche with their benzodiazepines and Rhône-Poulenc with the cyclopyrrolones. These series are their main "trumps" and they both arise from innovation and creativity. Arising from this there is a lot of more or less fundamental research to find something better. Up to now this research has yielded only "me too" compounds, at least as far as the benzodiazepines are concerned. When this happens with the cyclopyrrolones too, it will mean that rational approaches have failed.

Professor Andrews
I think perhaps that too strong a distinction is being drawn between the alternative approaches, between the so-called rational drug design idea and the approach put forward by Dr Messer. Looking through his last slide, I think that it is fair to say that most of the steps that he outlined are precisely the ones that everyone else has been talking about. Beginning with the belief that specific pharmacophores exist, and that we can take advantage of them, we try to determine the structural requirements for that pharmacophoric action in particular drug molecules, which of course is precisely the area talked about by Professor Marshall. We then go on to use the knowledge, that may be internal to the company, about a biological mechanism, which is of course the subject of many of the talks at this meeting. Finally, there is the synthesis of these molecules, and then their optimization, which Dr Messer described. He said that optimization is not research, it is a routine business. I would suggest that 20 years ago when Professor Hansch was introducing optimization, it was research rather than a routine business, and in 20 years' time I imagine that all the things we have been talking about here will certainly also be routine business.

Dr Messer
I agree with that.

Dr Ashford
We have discussed the optimization of an active series, once an active lead has been discovered. In my experience, however, many compounds are rejected from an active series because of side-effects and too low a therapeutic margin of safety. It seems to me that Professor Trouet's approach of drug targeting is a very good one, and perhaps we ought to spend more time on developing that end of it, perhaps getting more of our active compounds through to the clinic.

Professor Marshall
I commend the speakers for having used hyperbole and provoking a lot of discussion.

It seems to me that there were several misconceptions presented in the talks, probably on purpose. First, I think it would be a disaster to perpetrate a group of high priests on the medicinal chemists, people to whom they would come for guidance and leadership, to draw a structure and have it come out of the computer, and for the medicinal chemists to have to go back to the laboratory and make this thing dictated by some machine. That concept is so far from reality that it ought to be stopped very quickly. At best, what we can do is to help to cultivate the creativity, and help to make use of the insight and experience which people have garnered with tremendous labour. That is really the goal about which most of us have been trying to talk.

Secondly, we really are in the midst of a biological revolution. The information being obtained, in terms of molecular mechanisms, in terms of new things, is overwhelming. I am struck not by the fact that there is a lack of opportunities for therapeutic intervention but how to decide on which ones to put our money. It seems to me that that is really the big problem; it is not even a question of how to go about doing it. Being a "peptide person", there are 15 or 20 targets in the central nervous system on which I could put my whole group to work for the next 10 years, I think very productively. The question is which one do I try to make use of? Perhaps we are underselling slightly; I think we all recognize it, but perhaps we have not emphasized it quite enough.

There is the emphasis, for instance, on the non-steroidal anti-inflammatories: a Nobel Prize has been given for the mechanism of action of at least a large subset of that set of compounds. Certainly, I would not argue that the compounds were discovered prior to the mechanism but now, knowing the mechanism, it would be very easy to do some interesting things.

Professor Wooldridge

Obviously, I was trying to be provocative. Nevertheless, with some of the real problems that we have – I mentioned arthritis and atherosclerosis, which are here, right with us, and are very big problems – the biological and biochemical mechanisms are imperfectly understood. They are very complex, and I think it will be many years before the sort of techniques about which we have been hearing can really be applied. The problems are with us now: what do we do?

Professor Marshall

It is an imperfect world. However, it seems to me that with the revolution in immunology, our understanding of immunology and the impact of that, that we will not have to wait too long before there is a good insight into what to tackle, in terms of arthritis.

Professor Wooldridge

I hope you are right.

Dr Dearden

First, to follow on from Professor Marshall's comments about non-steroidal anti-inflammatories, we are one of the groups working on them. We have not particularly taken account of Vane's work regarding prostaglandins and so on in designing new drugs. We have started from the other end, by looking at existing active drugs, and have then proceeded to predict a receptor from that. Now that a lot is known about prostacyclin, cyclooxygenase and so on, we are in the process of tying in our projected receptor with what Vane has said. The point I want to make is we do not *have* to have a known receptor before starting to do this sort of work. Certainly, we have to have some known active drugs, but there is no need to have a known receptor.

Secondly, I confess that I was slightly unhappy with Dr Messer's emphasis towards the end of his talk on substructural units. What bothers me is the following: a receptor site does not recognize, for example, a methyl group, or whatever; it recognizes a certain collection of electrons in a certain shape and so on. Organic chemists, in particular, tend to think in terms of groups, where they should really be thinking in terms more of physicochemical parameters.

Perhaps I may illustrate this by one very small point. We tend to think that non-steroidal anti-inflammatories, as a group, should have a carboxyl group on them. Indeed, it is almost heresy, in some places, to design an anti-inflammatory without a carboxyl group on it. Just for "fun", as it were, we took a chemical off our shelves. It happened to be 3,5-di-isopropylphenol. We tested it, and found that it was a better anti-inflammatory than aspirin.

Professor Whalley
But, of course, it was probably more toxic.

Dr Wold
I want to discuss the concept of optimization which I think is greatly misused, here and everywhere else, in chemistry. Chemists believe that they can optimize things by changing one variable at a time. This is not true, and it is not true either in drug design. From what I have seen here, and from what I have seen in the drug industry in the United States and Sweden, this is the standard procedure. One substituent is changed, then another, then one fragment — and so on.

The problem is that if there are complex systems, as pointed out by Professor Hansch, this is a highly inefficient procedure which can mathematically be shown to be pseudo-convergent, and we get stuck with far lower activity than could be achieved, and moreover, we do not realize that we are stuck. We think we have reached the optimum because only one thing is varied at a time. This happens if, for example, the enzyme has flexibility and can change with the modifications that are made. Methods for getting round this problem were developed at ICI about 40 years ago. It is common knowledge in chemical engineering, but has not yet reached synthetic chemistry or drug design. I think there is much to do in what has been called "optimization", but which I call pseudo-optimization, by introducing simple strategies for varying several things at a time and evaluating the results in a proper statistical way.

Professor Whalley
One substituent at a time can be changed, but it is impossible to change one variable at a time. If hydrogen is changed for a metal, that has changed one variant, but that has presumably also changed the permeability, the lipophilicity and so on. Therefore, that automatically introduces several variables even when only one substituent is changed, does it not?

Dr Wold
That is not what I mean — that is a further complication. But already, if we just look at one substituent at a time and think that we are changing only one property of the molecule, even if it was so simple we would still not be optimizing

things. This problem is complicated by what Professor Whalley has pointed out, that the variables with which we like to reason, such as lipophilicity, electronic properties and so on, are our constructs. The receptor does not think in the same way that we do. We like to use these things, and the problem is that they all change at the same time – that is a further complication. What I am saying is that already in the simple case, if we just change one substituent, it can be shown that there is pseudo-convergence.

Professor Wooldridge
I believe that this is applied to improve a chemical process (originally by Professor Box, (Box, G.E.P. and Draper, N.R., 1969. "Evolutionary Operation: Statistical Method for Process Improvement", Wiley)) but I am unaware of the technique being applied to drug design. Would you tell us something more about this application?

Dr Wold
Once it is realized that there is a problem, that if one variable at a time is changed we get stuck, the simple thing is to change all the possible things simultaneously. However, the problem with that is that if the strategy is no good, we get lost – because man is unable to think about more than one variable at a time, with his normal ability, so-to-speak. Therefore, there must be some sort of guidelines (this is called "experimental design") about how to manipulate several things at the same time, regardless of the system being studied. This is used a great deal in process control where Box has devised several schemes, one of which is to go in a certain direction – but that works only if there are continuous variables, so it does not work in drug design. However, he has generalized these things to cope also with discrete changes, such as substituents – and there it works very well. I have not seen it used anywhere in the drug industry, except in places where I have some influence.

Professor Stevens
If I may touch on a subject which has not been discussed – that is, how to generate the most precious commodity of all, new lead compounds. I work in a group which is trying to do that in the anti-tumour field. Apart from doing all the scientific things that we ought to be doing, we have a very unorthodox approach which I would like to describe. It may be found to be appalling, but as a means of generating new lead compounds it is proving quite interesting. It is exactly the opposite of what is done in industry.

A known active compound is taken, and instead of trying to optimize and to improve it an attempt is made to destroy its activity. I can give one example which is relevant to Professor Hansch's contribution, in the di-amino-pteridine, di-amino-pyrimidine, di-amino-quinazoline, di-amino-heterocycle field generally. The biological interest in that type of compound is completely dominated by inhibition of dihydrofolate reductase. What can those di-amino compounds do in other areas?

We got into this field really by chance – there is a di-amino-pteridine called triamterene, which ought to be a very good inhibitor of dihydrofolate reductase.

In fact, it is a very poor inhibitor, but it is a very good diuretic – it is a commercial product.

We have tried to take really good di-amino-heterocycles which inhibit dihydrofolate reductase and put in all the wrong groups – in other words, put in ionic groups where there should be hydrophobic groups, hydrophobic where there should be ionic groups. This is a way of exploring new biological activities of di-amino-pyrimidines. We have had some extraordinary results. For example, we can take a molecule which is a fantastic inhibitor of dihydrofolate reductase and an anti-tumour drug, we destroy its activity as a dihydrofolate reductase inhibitor – and the product turns out to be a better anti-tumour drug than the original product. That sort of example illustrates a way of generating entirely new lead compounds in old chemical fields. I commend it to everyone as a possibility to explore in other fields.

Professor Whalley
Triamterene, as I am sure everyone knows, is of course totally insoluble in everything. It is the last compound that should – or would – be explored as a therapeutic agent. In fact, there was so much resistance shown to it being explored as a therapeutic agent that it stayed on the shelves for 10 years before anybody bothered to do anything with it. It now sells at least $1000 million-worth per annum. There is some sort of moral there.

Professor Wermuth
Dr Messer told us that if everybody uses the same biological screening everybody will find the same drug but it sounds like saying that if everybody knows the same words everybody will write the same book. Fortunately there are so many combinations that I dare say everybody will not think the same thing at the same time. Professor Stevens illustrated this statement with an unorthodox approach and I can give another example.

I am involved with psychotropic drugs, a field in which the three mediators serotonin, noradrenaline and dopamine play an essential role. Whatever the mechanism of interaction is, we can select as a target a multiprofiled drug which increases the serotonin and dopamine level and not the noradrenaline level. In this case the classical battery of biochemical tools can be useful and lead to a compound with an entirely new profile.

Dr Messer
I think there is never enough novelty in a compound. If a compound could be marketed within three or four years perhaps one can be more modest and follow some biological ideas only. But it becomes increasingly true that it takes ten years and more to develop a drug. In this context, biological concepts are relatively short lived. On the contrary, the chemical series which form the basis of the innovation, have a longer life. In other words I prefer to work on new series the industrial life of which are known rather than on trivial or biologically fashionable series.

Professor Roques

But one can do both, working on new series and also starting with a biological hypothesis. Furthermore I think it is more pleasant to work on new series with some biological hypothesis than to work on old series in order to get something new. From this point of view Professor Wermuth's idea related to neurotransmitters looks to me very promising and readily workable.

Professor Wooldridge

From the questions that have just been raised, I feel that Dr Messer and I rather over-stressed the realistic approach.

I would like to say that, certainly at May and Baker, we are very much in favour of a theoretical approach, tempered by realism, and that what we are hoping to get from this meeting is perhaps some guidance about how much further we should go along the lines that have been described. We also appreciate that university departments, I would not say go for the easiest problems, but obviously cannot carry out sophisticated studies on enzyme substrate interactions unless they can get hold of a nicely crystalline enzyme. It is rather unfortunate that in many of the areas in which we are obliged to work, this is not possible.

I would perhaps like to restore the balance, moving slightly away from all the cold water that has been flying around − and state that we are not quite as old-fashioned as may have been thought.

Session III

14 Syndicate Discussions

K.R.H. WOOLDRIDGE

May and Baker Ltd., Dagenham, Essex RM10 7XS, Great Britain

Introduction

Following the formal presentations which were intended to cover the spectrum of drug design techniques, the participants were asked to consider a number of specific questions. To facilitate free discussion, and to enable full scope for divergent views, participants were divided into four groups which were balanced as far as possible with regard to experience and disciplines. However the syndicate chairmen were deliberately chosen from different disciplines (biochemistry, pharmacy, chemistry, medicine) to enable them to guide the discussions in their groups from a different viewpoint.

To sharpen decision-making, time pressure was applied by allowing only three hours for the syndicates to discuss all the questions and arrive at firm conclusions.

The conclusions of each group were presented to a plenary session by the chairmen and were then compared and discussed.

Questions for Discussion

The groups were presented with the following questions.

A. Two of the major problems facing the scientist engaged in drug research are to generate new leads and to optimize active chemical series.

Accepting this, identify for each category the most helpful approaches in obtaining a new drug taking into account the advantages, disadvantages and chances of success.

B. For each category, select the two best approaches at the present moment.

Also identify two techniques which, in the opinion of the syndicate, will make the greatest impact on drug discovery in the future.

Findings and Conclusions of the Syndicates

The results of the deliberations of the syndicate groups were presented by the chairmen at a Plenary Session verbally and visually. Since it is impracticable to reproduce these in full, the author has collated and summarized the information to try and present a more concise and coherent picture and to avoid over-repetition.

Question: *Identify the most helpful techniques in generating a new lead and select the two most useful at the moment and the two which will make the greatest impact on drug discovery in the future.*

Syndicate 1

In summarizing the findings of Syndicate 1, Professor Rabin said that they had found this a most difficult question to answer and in general felt that the new technology would not make a significant impact during the next five to ten years. Three possibilities were pinpointed.

Firstly it was felt strongly that structural information about the target is of central importance and could be derived from a number of techniques including X-ray crystallography, NMR, and consideration of areas of hydrophobicity and hydrophilicity. Once this has been achieved, molecules can be designed accordingly. The problem is that the target is not always identifiable but nevertheless some information may be available by analogy.

The second approach is to take advantage of the identification of novel pharmacological receptors or biochemical pathways and substrates e.g. historically, steroids and prostaglandins. Unfortunately, this sort of information occurs in a random fashion and usually everybody has access to it. Therefore the key step becomes optimization.

The third possibility, which is a very realistic approach, is devising new and meaningful test systems, particularly in some of the important diseases like arthritis. The problem is that the new system although excellent in the laboratory might not be relevant to the human situation.

The syndicate debated the most desirable techniques at some length but the consensus view was that the development of a new biochemical or pharmacological test system is the best approach, both at the present time and for the future.

Syndicate 2

Dr Dearden indicates that his syndicate had had some problems with semantics including the definition of a "lead". It was eventually agreed that a lead is the demonstrated biological activity of a representative of a particular chemical class of compound.

The preferred technique is to start with a known enzyme or receptor structure and to design appropriate inhibitors or agonists. The problem is that few such structures are known but there is every expectation that this situation will improve rapidly over the next few years.

However quite often the structure and relevance of the substrate is known, and this leads to the possibility of the synthesis of substrate analogues or transition-state analogues.

Random or directed screening has some advantages despite the low success rate, and this must be linked with the screening of natural products although this might not be intrinsically random. Dr Dearden's personal view was that there is still a considerable potential for lead generation from natural products.

The chance discovery of specific new indications for existing drugs is one of the most prolific ways of generating leads. This requires a study of odd or abnormal responses shown by drugs in the clinic perhaps by a closer follow-up of the yellow card system.

The syndicate's preference was for what could be described as the biological approach, that is the design of drugs based on a knowledge of enzyme or receptor studies and biological mechanisms. Chance discoveries from existing drugs could also come within this classification.

Techniques which might lead to progress in the future were considered to be protein crystallography and ligand-binding studies.

Syndicate 3

Dr Ashton said that his syndicate felt that more fundamental biological and biochemical research should be carried out in the pharmaceutical industry because such knowledge could lead to major innovations in drug design.

In agreement with other syndicate findings, the advantages of the use of computer-graphics and related techniques are clear when the structures of the enzymes or receptors are known. However if these structures are known, many companies may arrive at similar products which could lead to patent and commercial difficulties.

The "new chemical entities" approach expounded by Dr Messer had some attractions because it should lead to novel areas which would be of obvious commercial and scientific advantage. The disadvantages of this and the variants of empirical or selective screening are that reasonably high capacity evaluation techniques are required which may not be available or relevant to the currently important diseases.

Another approach is to study "outliers", that is compounds which do not fit into a pattern of structure−activity. Some syndicate members felt that this information could be used to design new chemical entities. This could be related to Professor Steven's idea that active new chemical entities may result from dismembering an active compound and adding large lipophilic or hydrophilic groups in what might be regarded as all the wrong places.

The best available technique was thought to be based on substrate or receptor antagonists with empirical screening as second.

For the future, molecular graphics and some form of pattern recognition were pinpointed. It was felt that the use of pattern recognition to relate physicochemical parameters would not generate new leads but the application to structural parameters should be useful in the future.

Syndicate 4

Professor Trouet said that his syndicate clearly believed that the techniques of blind and/or intelligent screening should not be abandoned because they offer the advantage of finding totally new chemical entities. In the case of natural products, complex structures are examined which are unlikely to be synthesed by organic chemists.

Secondly it was felt strongly that drug design is only possible when the biochemistry of pathological states is understood. The necessary research is long, expensive and difficult but the chances of success will increase with time.

Another important approach is to take advantage of clinical observations of unpredicted side-effects from known drugs. This has the great advantage of being immediately relevant to man and is cheap.

Finally the synthesis of analogues of endogenous substances may be considered with a view to antagonize, mimic or induce selectivity. Screening is minimized and the chances of success are good provided that there is a suitable endogenous substance to work on.

Overall Results and Author's Comments

As a part of the exercise, each syndicate was asked to identify the most useful lead generation techniques and then to select the two preferred techniques. In Table 1 the techniques are listed and ranked according to how many syndicates identified them.

The preferred techniques were scored (2 for the first choice and 1 for the second choice) and ranked accordingly (Table 2).

Clearly the biochemical approach emerged as the preferred technique at the moment although it was recognized that this approach had its limitations when the basic information was not available. There was also considerable diversity of thought on how the technique should be applied at the present time and in the future.

The syndicates rated selective or random screening highly because of various factors such as past successes, the possibility of discovering entirely new active chemical classes or more pragmatically because with some medical problems there was little alternative.

The other technique in the preferred category was the synthesis of analogues of pharmacologically active endogenous substances even if their mechanism of action was not clearly understood.

For the future the need for basic research in the biochemistry and physiology of the disease was strongly emphasized to provide the basis of a rational approach using computer graphics and other developing techniques. One syndicate recorded pattern recognition as a technique with considerable potential.

TABLE 1

Syndicate discussions: identified lead-generation techniques

Technique	Identified by syndicates
1. Identification of relevant biochemical pathways followed by the synthesis of agonists, antagonists etc. as appropriate.	1, 2, 3, 4
2. Random or selective screening including natural products.	2, 3, 4
3. Observations on side-effects or new indications of existing drugs.	2,4
4. The synthesis of analogues of pharmacologically active endogenous substances.	1, 4
5. Intuition, experience and general scientific awareness.	1

TABLE 2

Syndicate discussions: preferred lead-generation techniques

Technique	Score
1. Identification of relevant biochemical pathways followed by the synthesis of agonists, antagonists etc. as appropriate.	8
2. Random or selective screening including natural products.	3
3. The synthesis of analogues of pharmacologically active endogenous substances.	2

Question: *Identify the most helpful techniques in optimizing the activity of a chemical series and select the two most useful at the moment and the two which will make the greatest impact in the future.*

Syndicate 1

Professor Rabin said that his syndicate felt that the QSAR approach was a technique which has proved useful in many areas. The technique also has the clear advantages of correlating a lot of information and of being more objective. However, it is very important to plan the synthesis of analogues to provide a rational spread of parameters so that the full benefit of the QSAR approach can be attained.

Computer graphic techniques are also very important because they enable chemists to visualize their structures and to see how they relate to each other and to receptors, and this must assist in optimization.

Another important factor is the possibility of conformational changes on the target receptor. If three-dimensional structural information were available it should assist in optimization, particularly in respect of selectivity. The disadvantages are that it is desirable to know something of the conformational mobility of the receptors and enzymes and this information is difficult to obtain even using sophisticated kinetic techniques. The overwhelming disadvantage is the necessity of having the target in crystalline form which is difficult in the case of membrane-bound enzymes.

Professor Rabin added the personal view that the modern technique of gene-cloning should make it possible to obtain large quantities of pharmacological receptors which it may be possible to crystallize and enable the structure to be determined. Already two of the subunits of the acetylcholine receptor had been cloned.

The syndicate concluded that the best available optimization technique is QSAR closely followed by determining structural information of the target to be used in association with computer graphics.

Syndicate 2

Dr Dearden said that his syndicate were clearly in favour of the QSAR approach, not only the regression analysis pioneered by Professor Hansch, but also others such as Free-Wilson, and multivariate techniques.

Prodrugs lead primarily to improved delivery and there are many advantages to this approach. However a possible disadvantage is the possibility of side-effects due to the introduction of additional moieties.

Targeting is the technique capable of improving specificity and a great deal of work is going on in this field. It is difficult but has considerable potential for the future.

Pattern recognition could give some information about the receptor which may suggest ways in which the active series may be modified. However it is usually difficult to map the receptor sufficiently precisely to enable this to be done.

Another approach which could not easily be defined was what was finally called "experimental design" although a better term might be "empirical design'. By this was meant the "seat of the pants" or pragmatic approach to optimization rather than number-crunching.

Dr Dearden said that the approaches preferred by his syndicate were experimental design and pattern recognition. Personally he was surprised that QSAR was not selected.

Syndicate 3

Dr Ashton said that his syndicate separated QSAR from SAR. These approaches often worked and are usually quick but the biggest problem is the availability of good biological data.

Prodrugs were felt to have advantages in possibly improving bio-availability and selectivity. Improved formulation could also improve bioavailability.

Drug targeting was felt to have the potential of achieving selectivity but with present knowledge may be of limited application.

The syndicates were in complete agreement that some form of QSAR/SAR is the best technique for optimization in a chemical series and that prodrugs or bioprecursors could be useful.

Syndicate 4

Professor Trouet said that his syndicate liked the QSAR approach because it seemed to be cheap, rapid, and it worked. However it is restricted to homologous series.

Pattern recognition has the advantage that it enables a wide variety of structures and activities to be studied. However, the results are difficult to evaluate and the chances of success are low.

The computer graphics technique has the advantage of demonstrating chirality and conformation but is expensive and still remains to be proved by the ultimate test of devising a drug which has been introduced into the clinic.

The prodrug concept is proven with high chances of success. A possible application which should not be overlooked is the improvement of uptake and transport of the compound in cells. This may follow from a study of the relationship of these parameters to the chemical structures in a series.

The syndicate concluded that the best techniques for lead optimization are computer graphics and QSAR.

Overall Results and Author's Comments

In a similar way as described for the previous questions, Tables 3 and 4 were prepared.

There was obviously strong support for the use of quantitative structure–activity studies for optimization of a chemical series, particularly in conjunction with a carefully planned set of analogues in order to provide a rational spread of physicochemical parameters.

It should be recorded however that several participants were most unhappy about the way statistics were applied by many exponents of QSAR techniques.

Computer graphics were also highly rated but there appeared to be no general agreement as to the best way to apply these techniques in practice.

Optimization on the basis of experience or "gut-feeling" was extensively discussed in several of the syndicates, but it was clearly not easy to pin-point the thought processes or principles involved.

Pattern recognition was highlighted as a preferred technique by one syndicate although in the present context and meaning, it perhaps could be regarded as a variant of QSAR.

Prodrugs, bioprecursors and targeting were perceived as techniques which might improve on the effectiveness or use of a particular compound but may not necessarily aid optimization within a series.

For the future, molecular graphics, topographical SAR and more sophisticated statistical techniques were considered to have the greatest potential.

TABLE 3

Syndicate discussions: preferred optimization techniques

Technique	Identified by syndicates
1. Quantitative Structure Activity Studies (QSAR)	1, 3, 4
2. Computer graphics based on target structure	1, 4
3. Experimental Design (Experience?)	2
4. Prodrugs/Bioprecursors	1, 2, 3, 4
5. Pattern Recognition	2, 4
6. Targeting	2, 3, 4
7. Formulation	3

TABLE 4

Syndicate discussions: preferred optimization techniques

Technique	Score
1. Quantitative Structure−Activity Studies	5
2. Computer graphics	3
3. Experience	2
4. Pattern Recognition	1

General View of the Syndicate Discussions

Although the syndicate technique has been used widely in other fields, there is little published on its use in the realm of drug design, and it may be useful to make some general comments reflecting the general consensus of the meeting.

The individual syndicate discussions were lively, wide-ranging and thought-provoking and provided an opportunity for all participants to make a contribution and to interact with experts in other techniques and disciplines.

One very obvious problem was the question of semantics. Such terms as leads, pattern recognition, and even screening tests had often very different meanings to the participants. In fact one syndicate spent a considerable part of their discussion time in deciding on definitions. This also made comparison of the formal findings of the syndicates difficult. Some participants found the three hour session exhausting yet not long enough and would have preferred perhaps two shorter sessions. However it was appreciated that time pressure was necessary to try and arrive at decisions.

All the participants found the sessions invaluable in that they were able to interact with individuals of various specialities, experience and countries, and the view was expressed by many that after the meeting they looked on the problems of drug design in an entirely new light.

15 General Discussion of Conference

CHAIRMAN: PROFESSOR OLLIS

Professor Ollis

At the beginning of the conference Dr Jolles indicated that the purpose of this meeting was to provide an answer to the very simple question whether drug design could be regarded as a method that could be usefully adopted by pharmaceutical companies in their search for new drugs. Of course, the two companies that he had in mind were May and Baker and Rhône-Poulenc. I believe that I can understand why those two companies decided that the time had come when it would be useful to bring together a team of experts who are associated with various aspects of drug design, and for you, as the audience, to judge, on the basis of the evidence placed before you, whether you would like to be associated, as medicinal chemists, with the search for new drugs when the direction of the research was determined to some extent by the principles of drug design.

Whether as a result of this conference you have become convinced of the usefulness of drug design will hopefully emerge during this discussion. I may even encourage everyone who is present here to declare at some stage whether they believe that drug design is a useful method, or a method which they, as employees of drug companies, would prefer the members of staff associated with other drug companies to use.

I think that we have the opportunity of evaluating the way in which this particular approach in the discovery of new compounds may be applied in the pharmaceutical industry. I hope that the discussion this morning will be directed almost entirely to providing a well-based answer to the very simple question put to us by Dr Jolles in his introductory remarks.

I would like to ask Dr Jolles and Professor Wooldridge to open the general discussion by indicating to us their personal reactions to what they have heard in the conference so far.

Dr Jolles

After being involved for so many years in medicinal chemistry, I would hate to decline your invitation to react to all the opinions, Mr Chairman, and I will express my views on the plethora of information and facts that have been presented during this session. My problem will, however, be that I only have a brain, whereas a computer would be necessary to analyse all the data.

First, I shall say that I have been quite impressed by the highly documented presentations of speakers such as Professors Hansch, Marshall, Clementi and Wold and by the sophisticated methodologies which they are now able to use; for somebody who has been watching the development of their approaches since the beginning, the progress achieved in the domain is impressive.

Now, if we listen to the conclusions of the syndicates' findings which, as you know, were working in four independent groups, it is striking to notice that there is a consensus among the experts who see the real benefit of these most advanced techniques as a tool for "optimization". Nobody suggested that these methods should be considered as a way for "lead generation".

No doubt, QSAR, computer graphics, pattern recognition, statistical analysis, are in the heart of what is commonly understood as "drug design"; no doubt, after what has been said, that now we face mostly *a posteriori* methods analysing, with the help of the finest "soft and hardware", an already existing discovery of medicinal research in order to understand it, to improve it or to correlate it with other facts. I do not want to minimize the importance of such approaches: however, it is for me a most important understanding from our discussions that today, at the end of 1982, these methods are primarily used to optimize existing knowledge and not so far to generate leads *de novo*. This will probably change during the next few years and I certainly did not turn a deaf ear to the more optimistically-minded participants, but in my opinion, for the time being, we still have to wait.

The methods which actually were suggested for generating new leads imply, in fact, analogies and correlations with known enzymes, receptors, substrates or, as Professor Trouet put it, the biochemistry of the disease. Therefore, I am slightly astonished that Dr Messer, who tried to be somewhat provocative with his overwhelmingly chemically-minded approach, could end his presentation without having to cope with the supporters of high biological input into drug design.

I understand that the syndicates' judgement parallels somewhat the attitude of many pharmaceutical companies: the previously listed biological approaches are expected to be the most valuable ones in the near future and whenever it is possible to rely on them, one has to rush to make the best use of them; in many cases, however, chemistry represents a unique tool for lead generation and it is quite noteworthy that this distinguished assembly of drug design experts did express, in the syndicates, such a positive opinion about screening, or more exactly about what has been called intelligent screening. Finally, I would like to say that the fact that no reference was made to toxicology and side-effects in all the reports and opinions surprised me in a way, specially because we do have with us in the audience many toxicologists, biologists and medical doctors. Drug design refers all the time to activity; we are most interested in activity, of course, but this is not the only objective when designing a new drug. To be useful as a drug, a molecule must comply with low toxicity requirements and I feel that this is a most important aspect which should be considered in drug design. Better delivery of drugs to the target, using drug targeting, prodrugs or formulation should improve their therapeutic ratio.

These are my first reactions, but I wish to be cautious in this extemporaneous review so as not to appear unfair towards the various strategies which have been advocated here during these past few days.

Professor Wooldridge

Like Dr Jolles, I think that my cerebral receptors are saturated by the wealth of information which has been presented to us. Of course, I agree with much of what Dr Jolles has already said, and will not repeat it.

It is clear that, as far as optimization is concerned, the QSAR approaches, computer graphics and so on are obviously regarded as being of very considerable value.

I have every confidence that with the techniques available to us, and with the developments that are occurring, optimization, while not exactly being automatic, at least can be achieved very rapidly by the application of intelligence and available techniques.

However, it is the lead generation aspect which interested me particularly. I do not think that I take quite such a pessimistic view over this as Dr Jolles does. Some of these techniques can assist in lead generation. It is very clear that the consensus of the syndicates was that the biochemical–pharmacological approach, a knowledge of biochemistry, pharmacology, receptors and so on, is essential. However, this worries me because invariably it will lead to the design of enzyme inhibitors and so on – leaving us with the problem of converting *in vitro* activity to *in vivo* activity. I felt that this is one of the main problems which the medicinal chemist has to face.

There are one or two other immediate observations I would like to make. I was very interested to hear of Professor Stevens' theory about his novel ideas on outliers. Also, I would like to know a little more from Profesor Clementi on why he regards partial least squares analysis as a technique of the future. The other thing that came through – emphasized particularly by Professor Rabin – is that there is no substitution for intuition, luck and serendipity. In other words, it is most important that scientists apply their intelligence, think laterally and leave no stone unturned to find new approaches to drug discovery.

Professor Hansch

I want to take this opportunity to say again how much I have enjoyed being at such a meeting. I have never attended anything like this previously, and I have heard many different points of view. I want to comment about two things.

First, I was shocked by the summary this morning from the different syndicates. There was a unanimous and widespread agreement on screening. I will go along with screening – but I take it for granted. If screening is going to be emphasized in this way, what about organic synthesis? Nobody said anything about organic synthesis. I would say that it is as fundamental as screening. Secondly, everybody looks at QSAR automatically as optimization. It is very obvious that it is an optimization technique, but, in my view, that is the least interesting part of QSAR. What I think is interesting about QSAR, and what we are trying to obtain from it is an understanding of the way in which small molecules react with macromolecules and macromolecular systems.

If we have understanding, it is hard to say what kind of things will be uncovered. I think that out of that understanding new lead generation ideas will develop. But I certainly do not want to say that nowadays we should push QSAR for new lead generation. However, as long as we get understanding, we will get new lead generation in ways that we do not expect. Let me give a trivial example of this. We have done a lot of work on partition coefficients in general anaesthesia, and see that if log P is about 2, and if there is a hydrogen-bonding type substituent, or perhaps a polar substituent, we can come up with a good anaesthetic as far as potency is concerned.

With that information − a very abstract concept − of a log P of about 2, and some polar group, we could write down all kinds of structures for compounds that have general anaesthetic value. The same is true for the hypnotics, such as the barbiturates. That whole class of compounds has a log P of about 2 and a polar group. We can devise all kinds of such compounds. However, there is not much excitement about the hope for a better anaesthetic. Thus I think it is a trivial but concrete example.

Let me give one other quick example that we have discovered ourselves. We were testing dihydrofolate reductase inhibitors on isolated enzymes and on two types of tumour cells, those resistant to methotrexate and those sensitive to methotrexate. A totally different kind of structure−activity relationship was found for the sensitive ones. One of the paramount things was that the lipophilicity requirements are astonishingly different. In the case of the sensitive cells, we had an optimum log P of about 0.8; in the case of the resistant cells, it was 6. That is a huge difference which is over five orders of magnitude. That is not really the kind of new lead generation being discussed at this conference and it will not help to cure some new disease. However, it provides a whole new thrust to research which I will think is rather different from optimization. I really believe, therefore, in the long run, that what we really want in science is understanding. I believe that is what QSAR is about. I would approach it from the point of view of getting insight and understanding, with optimization as a part of it.

Professor Ollis
Professor Hansch has pointed out that the analytical methods with which he has had an association over a number of years might be useful, not only in optimization studies but also in the discovery of lead compounds. It is an extremely enlightening point.

Professor Wermuth
Professor Hansch has made the assumption that all he needs is the correct lipophilicity and a polar group in order to have a general hypnotic compound, for example. In the barbiturate series there are some compounds which are

hypnotics, and other compounds with the same lipophilicity and the same polar groups which are convulsants. How can he explain that difference?

Professor Hansch
That is a good point. It seems that there is a very fine dividing line between hypnotics and convulsants, and if we get slightly beyond optimum lipophilicity it often becomes a convulsant. I was talking about the basic hypnotic activity. I am not saying anything about side-effects, toxicity and so on. But to get into basic hypnotic activity – again I am speaking of neutral compounds, not charged compounds – if there is a very polar group and an overall partition coefficient of about 2, we have seen scores of examples that fit that. I am sure that there must be exceptions to that rule but, as rules go in medicinal chemistry (which is not very far), I think that is as good a generalization as I know of.

Dr Lunt
Arising out of what Professor Hansch said, one thing that is very important is the way in which these methods of looking at the enzymes can help us with the problem, outlined by Dr Jolles, of the toxicity aspects. In Professor Hansch's lecture we saw in the DHFR series, in connection with trimethoprim, how the enzyme from the mammalian host was different from that of the bacteria. This selective effect of trimethoprim, which is very non-toxic, is undoubtedly related to that. It is a way by which, in the future, we may be able to approach this extremely vital problem of toxicity. Furthermore, as a practising organic chemist, I would say that I have been heartened by the general feeling of all practising organic chemists at this meeting that computers are our friends and not some sort of enemies.

Professor Marshall
I want to pursue Professor Hansch's point, perhaps in a slightly different way. The pharmaceutical industry has been very successful in generating new leads by a variety of different techniques. It seems to me this industry is very aware of the revolution in biology which is going on and makes it possible to take advantage of many new opportunities. However, it seems to me that we have either lacked the techniques, or perhaps the time, to listen to the answers to the questions that we have been asking of our systems.

Professor Hansch has emphasized that QSAR is certainly a method to try to listen to what the data are trying to tell us about the receptor. Similarly, I think that some of the computer-aided techniques, in terms of molecular graphics, can help us in the same way. Over 10 000 questions have been asked of the dopamine receptor. It is my contention that if we knew how to listen to the data, then we should be able to draw a three-dimensional road map of that receptor. This would enable us to do anything we wanted with new series, with new leads, for interacting there. If we think about the possibility of doing that, not only with the dopamine receptor but with many other receptors, this problem of side-effects becomes one that is tractable.

Professor Ollis
Professor Marshall, do you think that a knowledge of the details of the interactions that can take place at the dopamine receptor might lead to the discovery
of an important new drug at the moment?

Professor Marshall
Absolutely – because there is not one dopamine receptor but many. It is already
very clear from the work that many people have done over the past few years
that the dopamine receptor, for example, in the renovascular bed, is different
from the dopamine receptor in the pituitary, which is different from the
dopamine receptor in the CNS, for example. These differences are subtle ...

Professor Ollis
Can the differences be discussed in structural terms?

Professor Marshall
Certainly, the dopamine receptor in the renovascular bed has much more
stringent steric requirements than has the dopamine receptor in the pituitary.
It is easy to show that dopamine agonists or antagonists that work in the
pituitary do not work in the renovascular bed. It is very clear in structural terms
that there is a difference.

The only point I am trying to make is that these things are really exploitable.
I am continually amazed at the evidence that would allow me to say, for
example, that there are probably three, four, five or six angiotensin receptors
which we can start to differentiate. I am very excited about these possibilities,
but again there is a subtlety in the differences, and putting in a three-
dimensional framework is a real challenge.

Dr Ashton
Dr Jolles commented that the syndicates failed to identify the need for getting
better delivery of drugs to the target to improve their therapeutic ratio. In our
syndicate, within our category of optimization we identified prodrugs, drug
targeting and formulation. In our final conclusion on optimization, we included prodrugs as one of the better methods of improving bioavailability,
and possibly selectivity. I wanted to clarify that point now.

Professor Rabin
I think this was also dealt with in my own syndicate, and perhaps I did not
do justice to the subject. We considered this problem, and indeed we also had
prodrugs as one of our optimization methods. I might say, too, that when we
discussed QSAR we also considered the problem of toxicity. I did not present
it in my report because it was not clear to me what aspect of toxicity one would
try to minimize in the early stages – it is such a formidable problem. We were
certainly aware of it.

Dr Dearden
First, in defence of my syndicate, I would like to say that when we talked about
optimization we did not mean simply a maximization of the required response,
but minimization of the undesirable response too. Indeed, I would like to

emphasize that we felt this was probably the more important. After all, apart perhaps from consideration of expense, it does not really matter whether a patient is given 2 g or 2 mg of a compound. What *does* matter is what undesirable side-effects occur. These are extremely important considerations which certainly have to be taken into account in drug design.

Secondly, I would support what Professor Hansch said about the application of quantitative methods of drug design to lead generation. It is possible; it is, in fact, being done at the moment. Industrial companies should be looking very closely at the application of these techniques not only to optimization, which is a relatively simple sort of thing, but also to lead generation, which can open fields much wider.

Dr Withnall

Professor Rabin said that new biochemical–pharmacological test systems appropriate to the disease process will play a large part in future lead generation. I think greater thought needs to be given to what is the best possible test and this needs intelligence, on the part of the biochemist and the biologist. There is perhaps a danger in advocating screening, whether it is directed or random, because there is always pressure on the pharmacologist and on the biochemist to set up a screen, and then to screen as many compounds as possible.

It is not necessarily the quickest and easiest test to set up that will give the most appropriate answers. Even if the test is highly reproducible and absolutely reliable, it may not give the most appropriate information.

As a biochemist, I am obviously very interested in receptors, and in designing compounds to interact with receptors. However, the possibility needs to be taken into account that, to some extent, these are obvious approaches, and that intelligent people in other pharmaceutical organizations will follow the same lines.

Professor Rabin

I can give an example about new biochemical pharmacological test systems my syndicate had in mind. In connection with antibacterials, there is a huge effort on blocking cell-wall synthesis. But for a bacterial cell to grow it has to be able specifically to cut its cell wall in places in order to insert new material. Has anybody looked at that as a new test system, for example? That may be neither a very good nor a practical example, but I am not aware that anybody has either set it up or looked at it in detail.

Dr Wold

I would like to put forward a suggestion on this area of screening and of making new pharmacological test systems.

In my experience from other fields, the secret of constructing new and interesting tests is to go from one single number to many numbers. Let me draw the analogy with process control where there is now experience of this approach for about 30 years. Forty years ago, it was thought that it was sufficient to measure the pH, the temperature or something like that in chemical reactions, trying to optimize the reactions just by looking at what happens to the pH and thus increasing the yield. It was then realized it did not provide sufficient information about what was going on. Today, thousands of different probes are hooked up, giving out different signals.

I think it is the same with pharmacological systems. From what I have seen in the drug industry, it seems to me that pharmacologists are still preoccupied by trying to produce one single number that measures the activity. Perhaps they have another single number that measures toxicity, and so on, but they at least try to reduce the amount of data that describe the state of the system, in order to make it possible to analyse these data.

From the statistical and information point of view, an attempt should be made to try to characterize the system by as many relevant numbers as possible. There is no longer any difficulty in analysing these numbers. If we do not try to reduce them, but instead try to measure as many relevant things as possible, that gives us a chance to "catch" what is happening. This has been tried a little on pharmacological tests and in my experience it leads to an improvement in the efficiency of the test.

Let me draw the final analogy. People agreed many years ago that it is not sufficient to look at one rat because, even if it is possible to measure very precisely what is going on in that one rat, this is not precisely the same as what is going on in the next rat. Therefore, series of rats are introduced. It is exactly the same if there is one single test. That one test will never measure what is required very accurately because it is not precisely related to the final result. Performing many different tests is like having many rats. Intelligent averages can be obtained in various ways that relate efficiently to the final task.

Professor Clementi

I just want to explain to the meeting why perhaps the results of the second syndicate were slightly different from the results of the other syndicates. That difference was of course mainly because of my personal feelings about what QSAR and pattern recognition are. In my view, QSAR can be seen as part of pattern recognition. But that is probably not very important to everyone here. What is more important to establish, in my view, is that perhaps QSAR is quite often identified with the Hansch approach. If we regard the Hansch approach as the possibility of describing biological activities in terms of a number of descriptors, such as π (which is probably the most important), σ, steric parameters, or whatever, I am sure that this has helped quite a lot in the past and that it will continue to help in the future. The point I was making was that the mathematical models that are widely used in the Hansch approach, mainly multiple regression analysis, might no longer be the best possible tools to use to learn what are the relevant parameters to describe a certain, biological activity.

The other point, which has really astonished me during this conference, is the complete misunderstanding of what experimental design is in relation to pattern recognition. In my view, the mathematical tools of experimental design are exactly the same, but experimental design is something that has to be done at the very beginning, and it is the only statistically appropriate way of optimization by which it is possible to decide in advance what is the minimum number of compounds that has to be made to treat the data statistically and to get an answer to the question about what are the relevant variables. I was really surprised that this method is not yet widespread in all the pharmaceutical companies. That is the main point that I wanted to stress.

Professor Ollis
Do you have an example, Professor Clementi, that you could quote to us, showing that it is possible to obtain a different answer to the questions by using the QSAR technique, as compared with pattern recognition?

Professor Clementi
Unfortunately not yet. Let me say that I am very confident about the possibilities of the partial least squares method but we are really only at the very beginning of getting an experimental optimum design by partial least squares. I hope that in a couple of years we will have some relevant examples to show to people, by which to convince them much better than can be done at the present time.

Professor Ollis
Are you advocating the abandonment of the Hansch approach?

Professor Clementi
Not at all. As I said, I am strongly in favour of continuing to follow the Hansch approach, but perhaps no longer by multiple regression unless we are completely sure that those variables are completely relevant. In my talk, I tried to point out the pitfalls and the requirements of multiple regression. Now that we have available alternative statistical procedures that provide at least the same "goodness" of results, if not better, and do not have the same stringent requirements at the very beginning, I am suggesting that we continue to describe activities in terms of π, σ, and whatever we can think of, but perhaps not by multiple regression, instead perhaps using principal component or partial least squares analysis.

Dr Bost
I would like to comment briefly on the fact that natural product screening has been ranked, at least by one syndicate, at almost the same place as random screening. There is one case where drug design is not involved at all − that is when we are screening new fermentation broth. The microbes are not doing any real drug design. Yet, this appears to be a very important area since there is a consensus that new, novel biochemical substrates and pathways are of major importance in new lead discovery. I think the point was not sufficiently stressed, that natural products, or natural substances, for example microbes, could be of major importance in the discovery of new leads.

Dr Messer
Almost all the syndicates have considered that, at present, screening is one of the best methods for lead generation and, as an organic chemist, I am quite satisfied that Professor Hansch has emphasized that within this approach organic chemistry is fundamental. However, in spite of the many fields and

opportunities of organic chemistry, many very active drugs are heterocycles. I am surprised that considering screening and then organic chemistry, none of the syndicates had commented on this.

Professor Andrews

There are, essentially, just two ways of getting new lead compounds, one of which is by screening, of whatever sort, and the other is by analogy to some known basis. It may be the structure of an enzyme, or the structure of an endogenous molecule or of a known drug. If we put screening to one side for the moment (it is really not separable but let us put it to one side) then the basic approach to these problems by chemists is to make molecules that look like endogenous molecules or look like drugs. Most of the endogenous molecules from which we have to work − or many of them − include heterocyclic compounds. And, of course, many of the drugs that we already have contain heterocyclic compounds within them.

I would like to go on from that point perhaps to answer some of Dr Messer's remarks and to suggest that when we set out to obtain new leads from any of these methods, essentially what we do is to use our chemical intuition. This is what Dr Messer described as the ''intelligent'' screening approach to drug design. All that the techniques of computer-assisted drug design are doing is to offer a way of assisting the chemist to fulfil that intuitive approach, to enable him to quantify his problems, to quantify the comparisons between his molecules, to help him to design the set of compounds to synthesize in the first instance − which was a result of QSAR, with the development of cluster analysis − to help him eventually to analyse the interaction between his compounds and their receptors and, finally, to allow him to optimize them.

It is important to recognize that particularly the computer graphic techniques and other ways of understanding the analogies between substrates and endogenous molecules, or between substrates and drugs, will be very helpful in allowing us to develop novel strategies which will provide us with new leads. When we begin to think in those terms, perhaps many of those need no longer be nitrogen heterocycles.

Dr Caton

With regard to Dr Messer's comments, I think that there is a general tradition amongst medicinal chemists to work in heterocyclic areas, and rather to restrict their research to those areas. That is probably why, to some extent, the discoveries have been made in that area.

There is no nitrogen in prostanoids and they are highly active compounds, far more active than heterocyclic compounds. Of course, there are other possibilities, such as peptides and so on. We must be more alive to other types of organic entities which may well change the emphasis in the future.

Dr Ashford

I have been encouraged by this conference because it has shown me that there is a great possibility of taking knowledge of enzyme structure, for example, and translating this into drugs. But it has also led to the thought that we do not have enough effort in fundamental biochemistry within the drug industry.

It is all very well relying on universities and so on, but perhaps we need to put more effort in that direction, or into molecular pharmacology.

Another thing that has interested me has been the suggestion that by suitable carriers, and by the use of drug targeting techniques, side-effects of drugs can be reduced. I still feel that the major losses in an active series are due to side-effects. If we can target to the desired organ, we have a great chance of coming up with good drugs more frequently, and also of translating some poor drugs which are in current use into good drugs. There are numerous examples of drugs which are toxic, and which therefore are not used to any great extent. I think that we can translate mediocre drugs into good drugs by this technique.

Again, that leads to the thought that the drug industry must invest more money in this particular approach. In the syndicate in which I took part, we discussed the number of academic centres which do work of this sort – and they are not many, and obviously cannot cope with every need. Dr Jolles pointed out that the present carriers are too expensive and that the whole approach is not suitable for large-scale use by the drug industry. Perhaps, with more effort by the drug industry these new techniques would come.

Professor Whalley
At this very late stage in the proceedings, we have not really asked the fundamental question. To me, drug design means that we are looking collectively not for another "me too", which can be made relatively easily, or even a "super me too", which can still be made tolerably easily. We are looking for a totally new form of therapy, such as penicillin, β-blockers, H_2-antagonists. These are the real winners, I suspect, for which everybody is looking and hoping. This brings me back to the fundamental point: how do we generate that sort of lead? I would say we can get this in a minimal number of cases, on the basis of believing that we understand what happens biologically, making compounds which it is hoped will be appropriate, and discovering, through much toil, tears and trauma, that we have been successful – as in the case, for example, of the H_2-antagonists.

Otherwise, I can see no alternative in the majority of cases, until we have gone through this long transition to what I come back to calling "enlightened serendipity".

In order to make enlightened serendipity work, we have to find bright young people, give them first-class facilities, first-class encouragement, set them up in some laboratory or laboratories, and tell them to go away and get on with it. I see no alternative to this. It may not be a very acceptable approach, but I am sure that it is the only way, and history up to now has proven this.

I come back to my fundamental point, with which I suspect Professor Ollis may agree, that it is impossible to plan to make a fundamental discovery. If I am looking for a totally new form of therapy, for example, to combat arthritis, this would be a major breakthrough. We can relatively easily, in some way, make "me toos". All the techniques that have been indicated enable us to optimize these, including getting rid of the side-effects, getting the drug to the site and so on. This is not to denigrate any of the techniques; they are all difficult, but they are less difficult than the fundamental one of finding fundamental leads.

Professor Ollis

Having listened to those remarks, for which I thank you, having established your research group within a pharmaceutical company, how do you ensure that that research group is working as efficiently as it possibly can? How can you encourage them to discover a useful compound? Will you use the principles of drug design or not?

Professor Whalley

Insofar as the principles of drug design at any time are understood, and appear to be applicable – yes. But, clearly we are chasing a moving target in drug design, as we are chasing a moving target in any other sort of activity. For example, Professor Ollis and I, 30 years ago, spent many months, and sometimes years, trying to discover the structure of a natural product. Nowadays, we merely get the NMR, the mass spectrometer and so on, and in an afternoon we can tell what the structure of a product is. It is the same with drug design, surely; it is the same with any experimental scientific technique. It moves on, and clearly we must move on with it, or we get left behind.

Dr Dearden

I should like very briefly to summarize my feelings about this conference. We have heard, certainly, of the great importance of being able to quantify the data in a number of ways – quantification of receptors of enzymes, quantification of physicochemical parameters, quantification of activities and so on. I would hope that one thing that has come out of this meeting is the importance of being able to quantify.

Another thing that has come out of the conference is that it will be necessary in the future to try to make what perhaps may be called "conceptual leaps" to bring out these new compounds that we have been talking about, new classes of H_2-receptor antagonists, penicillins and so on. This is something which may be difficult to do by quantification; perhaps it needs more in the realm of "intelligent serendipity".

Therefore, I propose that we slightly alter the title of the whole meeting. Instead of putting the question "Drug design: fact or fantasy?", may I suggest that we say that in drug design we need to factorize and we need to fantasize.

Professor Tomlinson

One significant feature of drug design which has not been put down as a factor which I would commend to us all is that we design more meetings like this between industry and academia. I have been stimulated by this continued interchange between academia and industry. I have been challenged, perhaps for the first time, by industrial problems. That exchange of views can only lead to the better and more fruitful design of new compounds. I made a very rash comment to Professor Ollis before the meeting started that I felt that organic chemists had little to offer in drug design. Although I am characteristically rash, I am still not convinced that organic chemistry in the sense of synthesis, is at this moment generating new lead compounds. It is certainly optimizing.

As regards the meeting as a whole, it seems to me that the necessity for drug design is that the multiplicity of ideas should be acceptable to the company at all times. I think that it is essential that in the drug design programme flexibility of approach, the accommodation of new ideas within corporate structure, almost immediately following their proven ability in academia or perhaps even in collaboration with academia, needs to be a very significant feature of drug design. I am going back to something that Professor Whalley said in the syndicate, that if we are going to do research, as a drug company, we have to do it to the hilt. We cannot just "play" with toys. We cannot, for example, take a computer graphic system and play with it for a while; we have to go into the system, understand it and put good people on it − then ideas will be generated.

Of all the ideas that I have heard at this meeting, there seems to be no doubt that the computer graphics technique makes us appreciate drug molecules in a way in which, prior to seeing graphics techniques, I had never appreciated. That is the singular feature of this conference, that graphics will give us totally new concepts about the behaviour of molecules in space. I think that that is the evolution which will cause the second therapeutic revolution more than any other.

With regard to QSAR, for many years now I have not been an advocate of QSAR techniques − but I use SAR techniques. Many of the examples which have been shown this week have quite surprised me as they show QSAR can, in fact, not only optimize but also produce new compounds. This has been quite a revelation to me, and I think it has come about over the years because drug companies, in particular, have been rather quiet about the lead generation possibilities of QSAR techniques. I am very pleased to see that.

One other significant feature of this meeting, for me personally, has certainly been the responsiveness of the participants to drug targeting. I know that in summing up the results of the syndicates we have been saying things such as that it is not proven, it has a poor chance, or it will be expensive, but I think that is a very negative type of thinking. It is novel, it is not expensive to look at − we can just throw some money at certain universities or certain people, and I am sure that within the next five years drug targeting, whether through prodrugs, through conjugate systems, or moving on to the formulation aspects with particulate carriers, will significantly improve drug action. Significantly to improve drug action means to improve profits. It may not be drug design, but it will be a significant part of a number of companies' armoury in the future.

A final comment is to say that I cannot make a lucid comment on everything that I have heard this week. It is time now to go away for a month, or two months (as Dr Dearden was saying) and, after the first week, to wake up and start to think about things that have been said. It might be useful for the organizers to follow up, perhaps in one or two months' time, and ask specific people what they then feel about what they have gained from the meeting. That could be used to some benefit.

Professor Ollis

I shall now close the conference. On behalf of the visitors, I would like to thank Rhône-Poulenc and May and Baker for their wisdom in inviting the visitors to this conference. As a listener, I have learned a tremendous amount. One of the reasons why, as a result of listening to the speakers at this conference I have learned so much is because those who have organized the conference were adventurous in their choice of speakers. They brought speakers to this country from many foreign lands. I believe that I speak for everyone when I thank those speakers most warmly, not only for the quality of their lectures but also for the way in which they have interacted with everyone who has been at this conference. I shall not mention the speakers individually, but just say, on behalf of everyone here, "thank you very much indeed".

I should like to request, if I may, that our senior colleagues convey to the boards of their two companies our warmest thanks for the way in which they have provided the excellent hospitality which has been characteristic of this conference. In association with those thanks, I would also like to mention Dr Phillipson and his staff who have undoubtedly contributed towards the smooth running of the conference.

I believe, Dr Jolles and Professor Wooldridge, that when you conceived of the idea of having a meeting entitled "Drug Design, Fact or Fantasy?", you hoped that it would be an occasion when your two companies might derive benefit from the discussions; I wish both companies well. I hope you demonstrate by your future achievement that you have derived benefit from this conference − but may I assure those who have organized this conference that the visitors who have been invited here have thoroughly enjoyed the opportunity to participate in what has obviously been a very influential and important occasion. Thank you all very much. That ends the conference.

16 Conclusions

G. JOLLES

After the numerous presentations and all the discussions between the specialists of this Round Table, did we actually answer this question? Perhaps our query was somewhat Manichean and to take into account all the opinions expressed, our concluding remarks should be more moderate.

It is true that rational methods for the synthesis of new drugs are now widely accepted in medicinal chemistry. Within this discipline, the hardware represented by computer tools has taken giant steps forward in the last few years and the software can now rely on more and more scientific progress based on the new knowledge of biological receptors and mediators, on the demonstration of new mechanisms of action and on the recent discoveries of molecular pharmacology.

Many keyboards are now ready to play *accelerando* and *molto vivace* the great symphony of drug design and it means that this approach has become a *fact*.

The critical area of pharmaceutical innovation, the *de novo* lead generation, is unfortunately the area in which fantasy remains preponderant. Most of the methods discussed at the meeting are in fact primarily used to optimize existing knowledge, which is of course far from negligible. But the integration of physicochemical, biological, biochemical and pharmacological parameters for the accurate design of new molecules still remains quite exceptional. Of course, from the accumulation of new data and from rapid progress in research, one can expect that one day drugs may be designed by methods which are almost exclusively rational; of course the most optimistic believe that it has already become a reality but research scientists who are confronted daily in their laboratories with well defined therapeutic objectives know that this particular kind of drug design still belongs mainly to dream and *fantasy*.

Research scientists are naturally attracted by the intelligent and logical aspect of drug design but the conclusions of this Round Table do not provide at the moment the possibility of a strategy totally free from serendipity. At the Stock Exchange of Pharmaceutical Research, one should neither sell blue chips too soon nor miss the opportunity of acquiring new shares in time to become wealthy tomorrow; those who make the cleverest compromise will be successful. The advisors who participated in our discussions do not at the moment recommend selling the shares which have guaranteed the success of pharmaceutical research so far.

The last word will be left to Professor Hansch who did a lot for drug design; his equations enabled many chemotherapists to take their first steps in this field and his current research activities contribute, through more and more sophisticated means, to give a new look to QSAR. His philosophy may be summarized as follows:

"The two major forces in drug research are organic chemistry and pharmacology. It is the interaction of these two efforts that produces the fall out of 'screening'. The greatest possibilities for innovative drug discovery depend on an innovation in the test systems developed by the biochemists and pharmacologists: QSAR can influence the direction of organic syntheses but in the end it is the ingenuity of the synthetic organic chemist which produces the indispensable new compounds."

Subject Index